Modern Magic of
Natural Healing with
Water Therapy

Other Books by the Author:

Acupuncture Without Needles
Athletic Injuries
Athletic Taping Techniques
How to Develop a Million Dollar Personality
Stay Younger . . . Live Longer
Thirteen Steps to New Personal Power
Confidence and Power for Successful Living
Dynamic Laws of Thinking Rich
Talk Your Way to Success
The Prevent-System for Football Injuries

Modern Magic of Natural Healing with Water Therapy

J. V. CERNEY
A.B., D.M., D.P.M.

Parker Publishing Company, Inc.   West Nyack, N.Y.

© 1975 by

J.V. CERNEY, A.B. D.M., D.P.M.

Library of Congress Cataloging in Publication Data

Cerney, J   V
    Modern magic of natural healing with water therapy.

    Includes bibliographical references.
    1. Hydrotherapy. I. Title. [DNLM: 1. Hydro-
therapy--Popular works. WB520 C374m]
RM811.C47 1975   615'.853   74-23626
ISBN 0-13-595090-2

Printed in the United States of America

**Dedicated to
Martha**

A Word from the Author

Health is your most precious possession. To hold on to it your greatest necessity. To maintain it your most vital need. And, when illness comes—when non-health appears—it is your inalienable right to have a method at your command to correct problems as they occur!

HOW?

Through the *Modern Magic of Natural Healing with Water Therapy* . . . a method that can change the very course of your life as it did mine . . . a method as old as time, and yet as new as each surging moment of mind and body, crying out for life!

Are you aware that within you are the vital resources to restore health? Supercharged dynamos that can be leashed, sedated, or stimulated with water therapy? Do you know that you can direct and re-direct these forces by way of one of the cheapest and most easily available commodities in the world?

WELL YOU CAN!

All you have to do is learn how to use them! This book tells you how to restore your former vigor. It explains in simple language how you can live longer and feel better. You will learn how to cope with arthritic pain, backaches, hurts that you didn't know how to handle in the past. With the most primitive kinds of equipment (a lake, a stream, a bathtub, toilet or bowl, sheets, towels) you can achieve the magic of natural healing with water. No money is involved. All it takes is common sense.

Would you like to step into a health-world of your own making? Would you like to be able to use professional water therapy secrets revealed for the first time? Well, brought to you in this most revealing text is a harvest of hitherto hidden procedures. Along with my own 30 years of experience with water therapy I bring you secrets of those famous European doctors Oertel, Brand, Currie, Hahn, Priessnitz and Winternitz. From the Universities of Vienna, Berlin and Heidelberg come therapies little known in the U.S.A. Some of them from the Orient. Some handed down to me by my grandparents who were emigrants from Germany's Black Forest. All of them come alive and available in this book.

By using these long-hidden techniques you can now treat yourself at home. All of it laid out as easy as A B C. You will learn how to use that amazing sex stimulant called the *"T" Strap* and *"Fan Douche"*. You will learn how to use the greatest tranquilizer in the world—the method that brings you peace of mind and body—called the *"Rise and Fall Bath"*. You will learn all about *"Neptune's Girdle"* as *The* treatment for abdominal problems. You will learn to use the amazing *"Hip-Sitz Bath"* and the sacral spray that stops cold feet overnight. Neuritis, neuralgia, arthritis, backaches, headaches, and the antidotes for them are all in this volume and all you have to do is follow the text. All you have to do is use that wonderful common sense of yours—with the techniques outlined—and Nature . . . in its own miracle manner . . . will do the rest!

This book is not a scientific text. It makes no claim to be. It is primarily an organization of procedures to make it easier for you to treat yourself at home. It offers guidelines to follow. It opens exciting new routes back to a more healthful life. So read it with an open mind. Read it without bias. Develop your own little miracles as have I, and day by day your hurts will pass away. You too will become a believer in the *modern magic of natural healing with water therapy!*

J. V. Cerney
A. B., D.M., D.P.M.

CONTENTS

Contents 13

water
treatment
for the
HEAD

---

chapter

1

Subjects covered:

EARS	Deafness
EYES	Blepharitis
	Blurring Vision
	Conjunctivitis
	Styes
FACE	Facial Neuralgia
	Face Rejuvenation
	Eye Beautification
CRANIUM	Headaches
	Head Colds
MOUTH	Toothache
NOSE	Bleeding
	Hay Fever
	Sinusitis
SCALP	How to Grow Hair

```
┌─────────────┐
│             │
│    EARS     │
│             │
└─────────────┘
```

HOW TO DEFEAT DEAFNESS

Tommy G. went deaf. His inability to hear was coincidental with going to work in a tool and die shop. He blamed his job in the noisy stamping mill, but there are reasons for hearing loss other then noise. Hearing loss may begin with changes in the sensory areas of the brain. There may be foreign bodies in the ear itself (wax, beans, peas, bugs, etc.). Deafness may follow an overdosage of such drugs as Streptomycin. Hearing loss may come when menopause sets in. There may also be nerve damage from an accident or even from hardening of the arteries. Alcohol, or too much aspirin, quinine, or arsenic may bring it on.

Whatever the cause, lack of hearing presents a problem and Tommy G.'s problem turned out to be nothing more than solidly impacted wax. It refused to be loosened manually. Water therapy was begun as you will see in the following procedures. In three days his problem was over. He phoned in the middle of the night. He was all excited. "Doc!" he hollered, "that water therapy is really a modern miracle. I can hear again!"

To help Tommy, and to help you, here are the methods used. The procedures are excellent for all kinds of deafness no matter what the cause. You too will notice perceptible results almost overnight.

STEPS TO TAKE:

HOW TO TREAT THE EXTERNAL EAR
(3 ways to do it)

(1) HOT FOMENTS

Apply twice daily (morning and night), for an hour at a time. Fold a bath towel in eights. Saturate with hot water (115°F). Squeeze out the excess. Apply over the offended ear or ears.

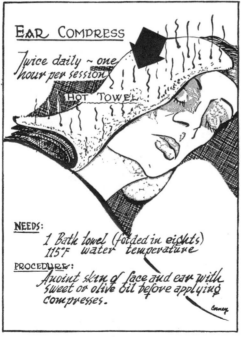

Figure 1

Alternate daily with the—

(2) STEAM UMBRELLA-TENT

This is best accomplished with a tea kettle. Get it boiling. Place the kettle on the table with the nozzle pointed at your ear. (Stay at least 18″ away). While seated on a chair cover yourself and the kettle with a blanket. Remain under cover for three minute intervals. Between steam sessions cool your face with a cold wet towel. (*Note:* Tommy G. found, by experimenting, that instead of draping a blanket all he had to do was sit under an old umbrella.) Repeat the contrast bath, hot steam on the ear three minutes plus cold sponging of the face for one minute, at least 10 times per session.

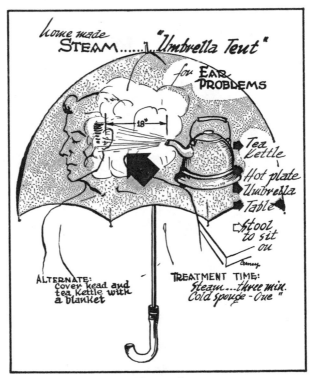

Figure 2

┌─────────────┐
│ *At-a-Glance* │
│ *Information* │
└─────────────┘

Other Non-Health Problems
You Can Treat with

DIRECT STEAM BATHS

Indications:

(a) *All painful problems* of the ears, nose, throat, face, tonsils, mumps, sore throat, laryngitis, earache, facial neuralgia, styes, boils.

(b) *Pelvic and anal problems:* hemorrhoids, vaginitis

(c) *Chest and throat* may be steamed for such problems as "colds", asthma, catarrh, bronchitis and influenza.

(3) EAR IRRIGATIONS

This procedure is simple and effective. If cerumen (ear wax) has become impacted (solidly wedged), it is wiser to start the loosening process with glycerin or olive oil. With a baby syringe, drop a half dozen drops of either oil into the ear before going to bed. Plug the ear with cotton. This prevents escape of the oil. The following morning irrigate the ear with a solution of bicarbonate of soda or table salt (one tablespoonful of either in a quart of hot water—120°F). Apply gently. Under no circumstance "dig" in your ears. As one of my professors once said,—"Put nothing in your ear smaller than your elbow." As the fluid exits, during syringing, catch the fluid and debris with a sauce pan held securely to the neck and jaw below the ear.[1]

─────────

[1] If your eardrum is known to be perforated DO NOT syringe your own ears. Let a professional do it!

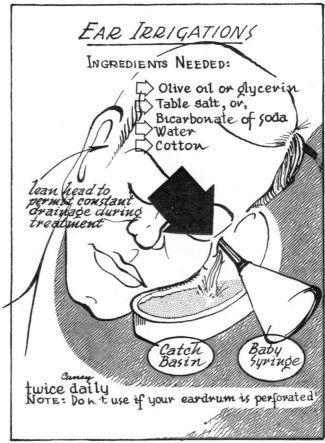

Figure 3

HOW TO TREAT THE
MIDDLE EAR

STEPS TO TAKE:

1. *DRY HEAT* is more effective on the middle ear if the involvement is mild. To accomplish this, place a dry towel over the offended ear area and lay a hot water bottle on top. Or, permit an infra red lamp (18″ away) to smile down upon it.

Other dry heat sources: bags of heated salt, electric pads, heated toweling or blankets, hot bricks. The degree of heat is controlled by the feeling of comfort and the amount of soothing relief which the warmth provides. Refuse to believe the danger- ous cliché that says:—"The hotter, the better." In fact the hot- ter, the "worser." Burns may occur. This is especially true for the aged and diabetic or those with circulatory problems. If you're past 50, be very careful about falling asleep during treatment.

Where Pain Is Intense:

2. HOT WET FOMENTS. Saturated folded hot wet towel- ing is applied over the affected ear. BUT . . . *an ice pack is applied just below and behind the angle of the jaw.*

Where Pus Is Present:

3. HOT WATER IRRIGATIONS into the ear with a baby syringe. Warm oil (sweet or olive oil) may be applied instead of water. Drain the outflow into a pan. Deafness and tinnitus (roar- ing and strange noises) often respond to heat in this manner. Hastened and improved results may occur with alternating hot and cold applications of water or oil. In Tommy Gaylord's case we added reflex therapy on the foot. Exactly how this is done is noted in Figures 4 and 5.

4. SPIRAL COLD PACK ON THE FEET. Fold a large turkish towel in thirds lengthwise. Saturate with cold water. Squeeze out the excess water. Apply spiral bandage from toes to middle one-third of leg. Re-apply cold pack as it warms. Apply before bedtime. Leave on after the fourth application. You will awaken during the night, throw it off on the floor, and sleep peacefully. Thousands of hearing cases have been helped, down through the centuries, in just this way.

5. COLD WATER TREADING is an alternative to the above procedure. For greatest effect run two or three inches of

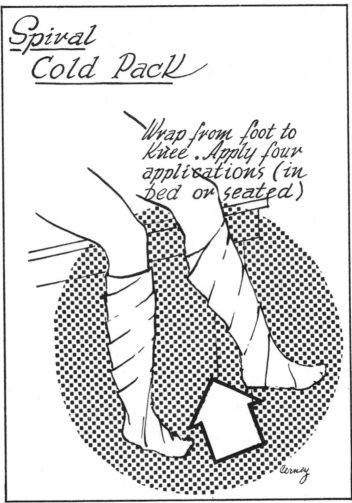

Spiral Cold Pack

Wrap from foot to knee. Apply four applications (in bed or seated)

Figure 4

cold water into the bath tub. Walk back and forth in it as long as you are comfortable. (The same may be done on wet stones, dewy grass, in a lake or stream.) Dry your extremities and either go to bed or get your shoes and stockings on and go to work. As you become more adjusted to this procedure fill the tub calf-high. This simple effective play-time not only gives you a physical lift but reflexly affects the ears as well. Do it! Note the results! You'll become a convert as was I.

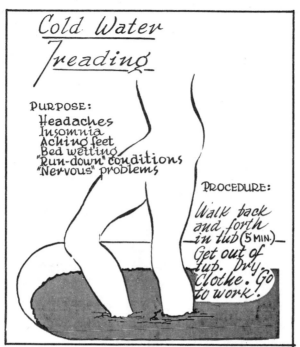

Cold Water Treading

PURPOSE:
Headaches
Insomnia
Aching feet
Bed wetting
"Run-down" conditions
"Nervous" problems

PROCEDURE:
Walk back and forth in tub (5 MIN.) Get out of tub. Dry. Clothe. Go to work!

Figure 5

At-a-Glance Information

Additional Non-Health Problems
You Can Treat with

COLD WATER TREADING

Indications:

    "Run-down" conditions (general tonic)
    Bed Wetting
    "Nervous" conditions
    Poor circulation hardening of the arteries, varicose
       veins, etc.)
    Tired or *aching swollen feet*
    Insomnia

> ## EYES

HOW TO HANDLE BLEPHARITIS
(Inflamed Eyelids)

As it would be for any proud woman, bald eyelids, for Gracie McB., were a catastrophe. Her eyelashes simply fell out. Her eyelids got red and swollen. She complained that her eyes itched, burned and watered. She said she couldn't stand the light. Headlights during night driving tortured her. Then came little ulcers on her bald red lids. They exuded fluids. During sleep the fluid got crusty. It glued her eyes shut. Technically the problem is called *blepharitis* and although the condition is different from a stye, the treatment is the same. So see *styes* a few pages from here. Gracie recovered faster then she expected by using the magic of water therapy. In two days she was back at work.

WHAT TO DO ABOUT
BLURRING VISION

Taking a cold eye bath was the daily habit of the English playwright, George Bernard Shaw. He said it kept his eyes from blurring. A cold eye bath may be achieved in various ways. It may be applied with an eye cup or with a cold wet foment where there is the necessity to relieve pain and chase away inflammation. To accomplish this effectively apply alternate contrast temperature:—hot/cold techniques as follow:

1. COLD WET FOMENT is used where pain relief is desired (see Figure 6). Replace the cold packs (layers of saturated toweling) *without giving them a chance to warm!* DO NOT USE

ICE[2] This treatment may be used for "black eyes" or after a foreign body has been removed from the eye. Continue local application for one hour.

    2. IRRIGATION with cold water is used if there has been a direct blow to the eye, or burning by acids or alkali. Follow with hot foments to relieve pain and absorb inflammation. Procedures may be accomplished with (a) cupping the hands full of water and bringing them to the eyes, (b) inserting the face into a basin of cold water, (c) pouring water directly over the face from a pitcher, or from a faucet in the kitchen sink.

    3. HOT WET FOMENTS (layers of wet toweling) are used primarily to improve local blood supply to the eyeball. This should be done three times daily where there has been actual injury or ulceration.

HOW TO CURE CONJUNCTIVITIS ("PINKEYE") OVERNIGHT

    You will be constantly astonished at your own success with water therapy. Each application will be a little miracle of your own making. This is especially true in conjunctivitis which means inflammation of the eye. A cold foment (wet toweling) renders almost immediate relief by chasing away an overactive local blood supply. Conjunctivitis is also called "pinkeye" because of its unsightly color.

    Julie R. had pinkeye. It was a bad case. Although pinkeye has many possible causes it didn't take long to determine why her eyes were watering, red, and itching incessantly. Her lids burned and smarted. She said she couldn't stand bright lights. After a night's sleep she would awaken with her eyelids welded shut. Her eyelids swelled. Little blood vessels in her eyeball looked as though they were going to burst. On-the-job pollutants were the

---

[2]False cataracts form when fluids of the eyeball freeze due to the proximity of ice.

cause. She worked in the office of a cement factory where the dust was thick. Here are the procedures that brought her dramatic results overnight.—

STEPS TO TAKE:

1. COLD WET FOMENT for conjunctivitis: Fold a small hand towel. Saturate with cold water. Squeeze excess out and mould toweling gently over *both* eyes. Cover with a piece of plastic (Saran Wrap) to retain the cold temperature. Repeat the

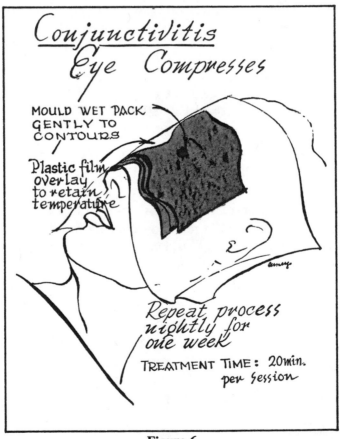

Figure 6

process as the foment warms. Keep repeating for one hour. After removing the wet pack, cover the eyes with a dry towel. Lie back. Relax. Eye tissues will return quickly to normal. *Added Note:* In conjunctivitis, repeat the treatment nightly for a week even though the problem clears up with the first treatment.

2. SCOTCH DOUCHE (spray) for conjunctivitis or iritis. Wrap your head with toweling in turban fashion, or wear a bathing cap if you want to keep your hair dry. Attach a spray hose to the bathtub faucet. While sitting on the edge of the tub bend your head forward. Turn on the cold water. Keep the spray going in circular motions as you encircle the face. Move from the outside in toward—but NEVER OVER—the eyes! Keep the spray head

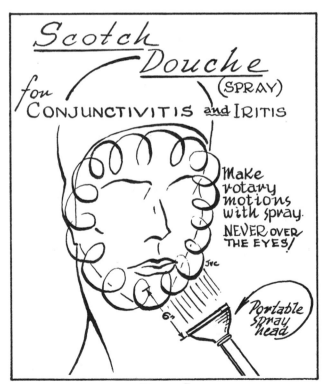

Figure 7

four to six inches from target. The force of the water should render a slight sting on impact. If it hurts, turn the faucet down. Be gentle. Repeat at least ten excursions around the face. Pat your face dry. Lie down in bed. Cover the eyes with a soft cloth saturated with cold water. Note the pleasurable soothing effect after just 30 minutes of this treatment. After a night's rest, your eyes—in uncomplicated cases—will feel completely rejuvenated. There are additional fringe benefits. You will not only find yourself seeing better then before but (a) *your complexion will improve,* (b) *your hair will start returning to its normal color if it has begun to turn gray.* I know! It happened to me!

HOW TO CURE STYES
IN RECORD TIME

Styes are found on the edge of eyelids. They begin when a sebaceous gland becomes inflamed, and resolve by "coming to a head." Jenny J. had a stye. She came to the office complaining of "something in her eye." It felt that way. Her eyelids were red and watering. Quick relief came by using the following:—

STEPS TO TAKE:

1. COLD WET FOMENTS (tap water temperature only. Absolutely NO ICE!)

Apply treatment over *both* eyes even though just one seems to be involved. Congestion, itching and hurt will stop. If the stye looks as if it is "coming to a head," replace the cold foment with a hot foment over the affected eye *only until the pus pocket opens.* Keep both eyes closed as you have someone wash the pus away. Cleanse gently via the following method:—

2. EYE IRRIGATIONS

At all times, irrigations are meant to cleanse, soothe, medicate or even lubricate. Irrigations hasten suppuration. They promote healing and are most effective at approximately 100°F to 120°F depending on the part being treated. The flow of water from a syringe, or pitcher, should be uninterrupted. It should be steady and comfortable to receive. *Precautions:–* (1) *Do not apply pressure on the eye at any time,* (2) *Shield the uninvolved eye if only one is being treated,* (3) *In applying the irrigation, apply from the corner of the eye outwardly toward the ear,* (4) *Cover the ear to keep contaminated fluid from flowing in.* (This may be circumvented by catching the flow with a pan at the corner of the eye.) (5) *Wash hands before and after an eye irrigation,* (6) *Dry the eyes with sterile gauze.* Follow the treatment with cold water foments over both eyes.

3. CHECK FOR LOCAL INFECTION

In the case of the stubborn stye there is, more often than not, an infection of one kind or another in the head, neck or shoulder. Where such an infection (tooth, ear, etc.) exists, see your doctor.

4. PROPHYLAXIS

A. Stop using your eyes so much (close reading, etc.)
B. Slow down! Take it easy! The world will still be going around after you and I are gone.
C. Add Vitamins A, C, and D to your diet. Eat plenty of fresh fruits and vegetables.

FACIAL NEURALGIA
(Tic Douloureux) and What to Do

**Comptometer Operator
Stops Facial Pain**

In the middle years, about age 50, a pesky pain called *tic douloureux* makes an appearance. More often then not it is a woman who gets it and severe pain hits one or more branches of the trigeminal nerves in the face. Melanie C., aged 52, a comptometer operator, developed this problem. She had no warning. Suddenly, there it was one morning while she was preparing breakfast. It was a lightning-like stabbing pain that didn't last too long. It started on one side. Two days later it was ripping through both sides of her face. At first the pain was momentary. It was gone for a week the first time around. Then it reoccurred and went away for a month. Then the periods started getting shorter. When something, or someone, touched parts of her face or mouth—a wisp of hair, a kiss, etc.—it precipitated another "attack." If you are having a true facial hypersensitivity in one part of your face, there will probably be numbness in another part. For Melanie, her home treatment was simple. Here's what she did:—

STEPS TO TAKE:

1. ICE RUB ON KEY FACIAL POINTS. The secret of this treatment is to quell the "hot" hurt areas along the nerves' branches. To do this effectively take an ice cube (wear gloves) and start a gentle rotating motion over the key areas indicated in Figure 8. Follow in numerical order:—(1) midpoint over the eyebrow, (2) below the eye at midpoint, (3) just under the cheekbone lateral to the eye, (4) beside the wing of the nose, (5) between lower lip and chin, (6) temples, (7) just in front of the ear, (8) back of the neck.

In treating the back of the neck, make rotary motions with the ice from skull to shoulder on either side of the spinal column. Move right on up into the hairline. Keep the ice moving. Repeat procedure for one minute. Then place the warm palm of your hand on the cold area. Hold for ten seconds and repeat the ice performance. Alternate at least three times or until the pain subsides.

Melanie called me hours later. There was an element of surprise was in her voice. She reported that not once had she had a reoccurrence.

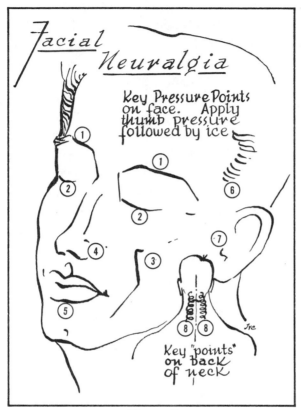

Figure 8

FACE REJUVENATION

**YOUR FACE . . . and How You Can
Use Water Therapy to Stay
Looking YOUNGER. . . LONGER!**

Her parents called her Dawn. From the start she was gorgeous. As a baby, she won photo contests. As a teenager, she won beauty contests. As an adult, she was even more lovely as she matured. Dawn C. was one of those fascinating women who takes her pick of suitors. This she did. As a member of the jet set, her beauty jumped out at you from fashion magazines, society pages and Sunday supplements. Then suddenly it was gone. Dawn came home. I didn't recognize her when she walked into my office. This exquisite beauty, this comely, shapely queen was no longer the Dawn Correlle whom once I knew. This was an old bag and the story she unfolded made me shiver. There's no need to tell you the dramatic details but the key to it all was *change-of-life* and self-indulgence.

It apparently hit Dawn like a bomb. Ugly hair grew on her chin and upper lip. Her skin was dry, flaky, gray, furrowed. Vitality flattened as did her chest. She'd already tried the beauty clinics that dot Europe. She went the gamut from estrogen shots to face-lifting and the story remained the same. She was living a personal hell some women go through at this time of their lives. It affected her personality. Something *had* to be done and I suggested the magic of water therapy. In her urgency she almost screamed at me—"Well, what are we waiting for?" We didn't wait. Treatment began. Within a month she looked and felt 20 years younger.

FIVE-POINT PROGRAM FOR LOVELIER SKIN, EYE BEAUTIFICATION, RELEASE FROM TENSIONS AND IMPROVED HEALTH

STEPS TO TAKE:

1. INTESTINAL LAVAGE

Always remember that *external beauty begins inside!* The body must be cleansed and Dawn C. was sick inside. In facial rejuvenation internal baths are vital and should be administered twice daily, two quarts of liquid per session. Because the intestinal lavage plays such a vital role, I want to take a little further space to explain it.

THE INTESTINAL LAVAGE OR
INTERNAL BATH OR ENEMA
(and Its Importance to You)

Internal baths are also known as enemas, irrigations, or internal lavage. There are five kinds. Each has a purpose as follows and you can use them to help yourself in achieving health as well as facial rejuvenation. The five kinds of enemas are:—(1) *Cleansing enema,* (2) *Retention enema,* (3) *Carminative,* (4) *Nutrient,* and (5) *Colonic irrigation.*

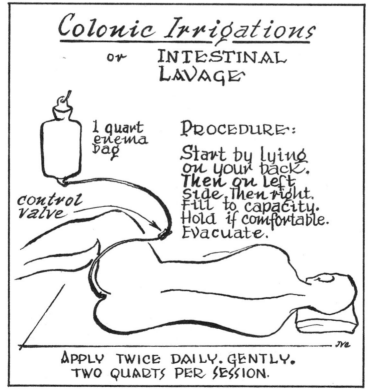

Figure 9

Cleansing enemas soften the feces, step up peristalsis and promote evacuation of the bowels. *Retention enemas,* even while softening the feces, soothe and lubricate the rectum and lower bowel. *A carminative enema* is designed to help get rid of gas. *Nutrient enemas* provide nutrition as indicated in the name. They instill liquid food into the bowels where it is absorbed through the bowel's inner lining. *Colonic irrigation* also does this with an added plus. It *flows constantly in and out at will.* Waste that has long been locked in the bowel comes loose and passes out.

How Should Internal Baths Be Given? In What Position?

To administer an internal bath efficiently, start by lying on your left side. This may be done in the bathtub, if you are small enough, or on a carpet on the bathroom floor. Bring the knees up. With your head resting comfortably on a pre-arranged pillow, lubricate your anus with shaving cream, soap, cold cream or vegetable shortening (avoid petroleum jelly). Insert the tip of a medium-size, flexible anal syringe. Water bottle should be above the level of the body. The water temperature should be 98.6°F unless otherwise indicated in the text. Before permitting the flow of water to ascend into the colon be sure to let the tube flow into the toilet or wash bowl to remove all air.

Administer an enema slowly. Open the metal lock on the rubber hose and keep your fingers in control. Permit free flow. Close off when necessary. Rest. Over a period of four or five minutes the water flows in gently by gravity. Your belly may challenge the flow. Should cramps occur from too much stimulation of the bowel or surrounding tissues, stop the flow. Close the valve or pinch the hose. Wait. If everything relaxes down there, permit the balance of water to flow in. If you do not have a great demand to expel the fluid just remain on your left side a moment. In this position, manipulate your left abdomen with the finger tips of your right hand. Stroke up toward the rib cage with little circular motions. You will hear and feel gurgling. Good! Now lie on your back. Repeat the stroking process on your abdomen from left to right. Then roll on your right side. Gently work the fluid from the rib cage down toward the thigh. If you get this far on the first trip you have done wonderfully well.

If you experience great discomfort and have to unload, remove the syringe, hold a soft towel against your anus, get up, sit on the toilet and evacuate. Repeat the process. This time, if there is discomfort, and you desire to unload before the enema bag is empty, pinch off the irrigator, knead your abdomen until the desire goes away.

What to Look for if There Is Discomfort During Application

Where the bowel is tender—from any cause—where it is packed or involved by diverticuli, stricturing or even ulcers, there may be severe pain when taking an internal bath. Where any of this exists—and pain occurs upon administering the enema—be aware that (a) *you now have proof positive of the very necessity for the irrigation,* or, (b) *your solution may be too cold* and you are causing additional stricturing or contraction of the bowel, (c) *you are permitting too rapid, or strong, a flow,* (d) *you are irritating the anus with too large, or too stiff, or too long a syringe,* (e) *you may be in a strained and uncomfortable position,* (f) you need consultation with your physician. *Note:* Stop all internal irrigations after the bowels regulate and become regular in movement.

2. DIETARY SUPPLEMENTATION

This is mandatory to remedy the tragedy of bad eating habits. To help yourself back to health, discontinue the eating of all pastries and sugars. Eliminate all alcoholic beverages and soft drinks. Cut meat consumption to a minimum and dine mostly on fresh fruits and vegetables. Add Vitamins A, C, D, and E to your diet. (Your local health store supplies them.) Use vitamins ONLY of organic origin!

3. STEAM AND COLD TECHNIQUE ON FACE (Review Figure 2)

4. EYE-BEAUTIFICATION WATER BATH

Here is an external lavage that not only helps the skin by acting as an astringent but also clears the eyes and improves sight. Railroader Calvin K. thought he was losing his sight as well as the youthful looks of which he'd been so proud for so many years. To prevent further erosions, he was instructed on scrubbing his face with an up and down motion from jaw to forehead with a rough towel. After the scrub, he was instructed

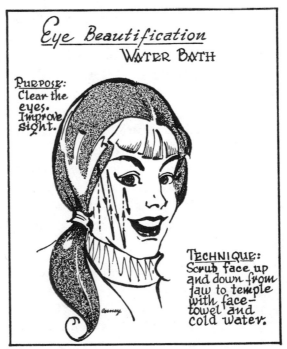

Figure 10

to rinse his face with a cold water contrast bath. To this was added the *Scotch Douche* (Review Figure 7) spray on alternate days. Calvin followed instructions to the "t." It worked! In a matter of weeks, his sight improved. Today, Calvin is no longer thinking about retiring. With his "youth" still under control he continues to hold down his job and be a man-about-town.

5. COLD WATER TREADING (daily—Review Figure 5)

**Age Is a Condition
of Mind over Matter**

In advising Dawn C. about the fountains of youth within herself that she could turn on at will, she was instructed on taking advantage of reflexes and additional Chinese acupuncture points. (See my book.[3]) By using these dynamic "points" properly you can actually push back the years. If it's facial rejuvenation you want, you can utilize additional magic pressure points on the face by pressure of thumb and/or ice cube.

HEAD

**HOW TO OVERCOME HEADACHES
AND BE FREE OF PAIN**

Pain in the head is a symptom common to many illnesses. It may be in one or more portions of the head and have one or more

---

[3]Cerney, J.V., *Acupuncture Without Needles*, Parker Publishing Co., West Nyack, N.Y., 1974.

reasons why it is there. Some pains come from outside the skull. More often then not their cause lies in the abdomen.

It was like that with Katie E. Katie is an older woman. She's an elderly physical therapist at a children's clinic for cripples. This lovely silverhaired lady started to have head pain.

Her headaches started at the base of the skull. A constricting band developed around her head until the pain was so bad she vomited. After vomiting there was temporary relief. Then it started up again. The doctor at the hospital said she had "migraine." Another pronounced it as neuralgia of the scalp. Neither examined her. Neither enquired into her life, her activities, her preoccupation with other people, or about her going without food and sleep. Both doctors prescribed that pain-mask called aspirin. No results.

That's when I first saw Mrs. E., examined her, and started her on the modern magic of water therapy. It proved to be the magic that not only promptly stopped the headache but helped her return to her usual vivacious self. Here's the technique:—

STEPS TO TAKE:

1. LOCAL FAN DOUCHE (on feet only)

My grandfather called this method *"faecher."* It's the German word for fan douche and he always used a garden hose to apply it. By turning the nozzle it produces a spray. The moment a cold fan douche is applied to the soles of the feet an amazing physiological reaction takes place. Excess blood is drawn out of the brain, and headache—from congestion—is relieved almost immediately. Apply for *one minute only*! Follow with massage of neck and shoulder muscles and a rest in bed.

> *Note: A cold fan douche applied to the neck, chest, and back, results immediately in deeper breathing, thus making it valuable in treating problems of the lungs. When the fan douche is applied to the abdomen, it stimulates the bowels. The liver, stomach, and spleen function better. When applied to the low back and tailbone, sex life is revitalized.*

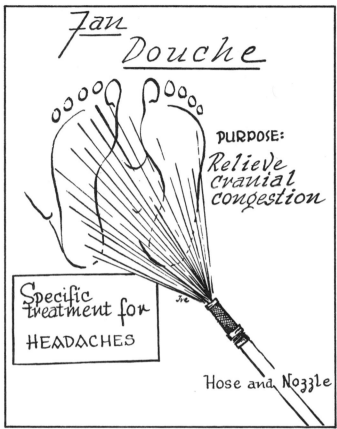

Figure 11

2. COLD HIP-SITZ BATH

Permit two inches of warm water (90°-95°F) to flow into the bath tub. Sit in it. Turn on the cold water. Permit it to run until water level is umbilicus-high. It's exactly at this point that the sitz bath is ended! Get up! Rub down with a coarse dry towel. Follow this immediately with muscle massage.

3. MUSCLE MASSAGE

The first necessity after water therapy (fan douche and cold hip-sitz bath) is gentle massage of the muscles to relieve their tension. Start with massage of the neck and shoulders. At first, these muscles will hurt. You will find them tight, unresponsive, some of them with knots in them. Under your, or a friend's, adept fingertips this will subside. Now massage deep in the abdomen and over the solar plexus (just below the tip of the breastbone). Now move on to my next professional secret for relieving headaches.

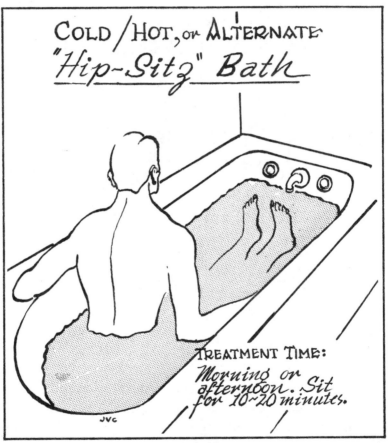

COLD / HOT, or ALTERNATE
"Hip-Sitz" Bath

TREATMENT TIME:
Morning or afternoon. Sit for 10~20 minutes.

Figure 12

4. STROKING THE CAROTID ARTERY

See Figure 13. Note position of the hand. To stroke the

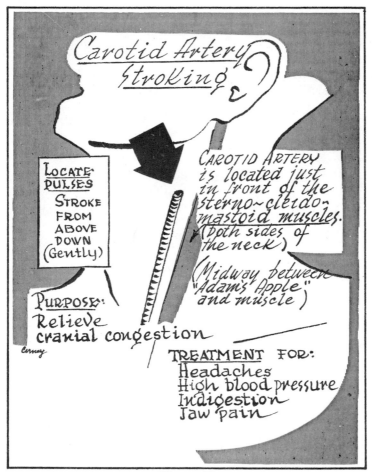

Figure 13

carotid arteries quickly and efficiently, stroke from the jawbone down to the base of the neck. Thumb on one side, four fingers on the other. Stroke gently. Brain congestion stops under this procedure. The valuable asset here is that the *carotid sinus*, the self-starter, is stimulated. Stroking this area also innervates what the Chinese call the *Stomach Meridian* and the autonomic nerves in this area. As a result, headaches due to cranial congestion, indigestion, high blood pressure, or even emotions are alleviated. Follow this now with an—

5. ICE BAG ON TOP OF HEAD AND HOT PACK ON BACK OF NECK

Place a cold wet turkish towel foment on the abdomen.

**Alternative Procedures for
Getting Rid of Headaches:**

A. *WATER TREADING* (cold), (Review Figure 5). One minute.

B. *HANDS IN BUCKET OF COLD WATER*. Procedure: three minutes in and one minute out. Repeat process at least four times or until the headache subsides.

C. *INTERNAL LAVAGE* (Review Figure 9) to cleanse bowel.

D. *AVOID OVER-EXERTION!* Rest! Drink water copiously till the kidneys are flushed out. Where a headache persists due to overstrain or fatigue, very hot coffee may be drunk but *take no other drug.* If headache continues, see your physician. With the above program there are no complications from treatment. Headaches are relieved almost immediately. Mrs. E.'s headaches were solved in a matter of hours and it will probably turn out the same way for you.

HOW TO STOP THAT AGGRAVATING "HEAD COLD"

The George Smyth family in our neighborhood had the runningest noses, the wateriest eyes, and the most stuffed-up heads I'd ever seen. That's the way it was until they started using water techniques. There are a number of approaches to "head-colds" on which they were instructed to conquer their problem. For the Smyth family—and for you—here's a stay-on-your-feet procedure for those who have no time to be sick in bed. Any or all of the five following techniques may be used depending on time, place, and occasion.

STEPS TO TAKE:

1. SPONGE-DOWN TECHNIQUE

In the nude, stand ankle-deep in cold water in the bathtub. Bend over. Dip your sponge. Systematically apply it from below up in long sweeps. Do the entire body. Do it quickly, efficiently. Then, *without drying* yourself, wrap up in a dry sheet and get into bed. Keep warm. Repeat at 60-minute intervals. After the

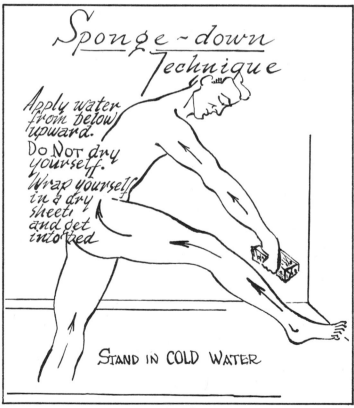

Figure 14

sixth sponging, take a cold shower, rub down briskly, don warm clothing and move around with your usual duties. The Smyths all use this method. It's fast, effective, and cuts down the misery time of a head-cold. It stops that stuffed-up feeling because the sinuses let loose.

2. SCOTCH DOUCHE TECHNIQUE

Morning: Run a sharp cold spray up and down your spinal column. (Spinal column ONLY!) Wrap yourself in a dry sheet *without drying* and get back into bed.

Afternoon: sharp cold spray on the *front of the body ONLY!* Wrap self in a blanket or sheet and get back into a warm bed.

Evening: same on *arms and legs ONLY*. Repeat the process for a couple of days. You'll be glad you did.

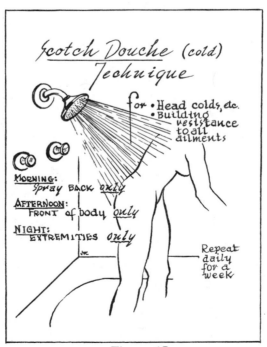

Figure 15

SPECIAL NOTE: With both the sponge-down and Scotch-Douche techniques you will experience a pleasant warmth stealing over you. You'll get drowsy. Take advantage of this natural phenomenon. Each time you accomplish this with the magic of water therapy you will look forward to the next treatment. By the third sponging you will begin to sweat. Poisonous body waste will flow out through the pores. Your nose will begin to flow if you respond normally. Let it out. Let it ALL out but DO NOT BLOW YOUR NOSE. Blowing only complicates the infection and drives the bacteria up into the eustachian tube to the ear. Drip dry. Blot gently. By the third day of this treatment you will feel like a million if your body reactions are normal. Stick to a liquid diet. Fast on soup and ginger ale. DO NOT drink milk.

3. FULL-TUB TECHNIQUE

For those who hate showers and can't stop to rest in bed the cold-tub procedure may be used. Here's how:—Fill bathtub with

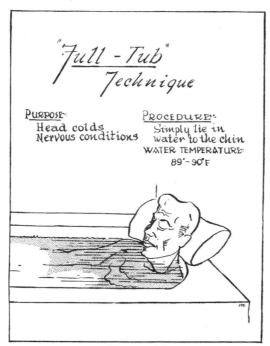

Figure 16

two inches of tepid water (85°-90°F). Lie down in it after turning on the cold water. Lie back. Relax. As the cold flows in, you will experience changes within you. Relaxation is one of these changes. When the water gets as high as your chin, reach over and turn it off. Stay in position for 20 minutes. Repeat the process morning and night. This worked so well for George Smyth Sr. that he went around the neighborhood telling how "I knocked my cold in the head just resting in the bathtub."

4. ICE CUBE TECHNIQUE

Apply this time-honored method twice daily. Use an ice cube (or the bottom of an ice-cold bottle). Apply the ice cube to the fat pad of the big toe with rotary motions. Note the pinpoints of pain you locate as you rub. Massage these areas until the pain recedes. Supplement this procedure with fresh orange juice

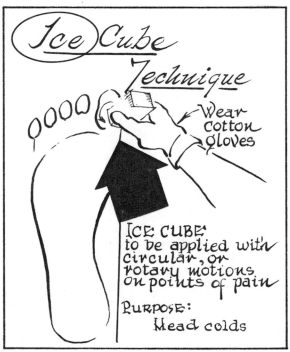

Figure 17

orally (all day long). Concentrated vitamin C tablets or lozenges may be used to supplement the diet.

5. THE WET "X" PACK

The wet "X" pack, as an antidote to the head cold, is an heirloom in my family. From my grandfather I pass it on to you. Here's how to apply it:—Fold a single bed sheet lengthwise into eighths. Soak sheet in a bucket of cold water. Place free end of

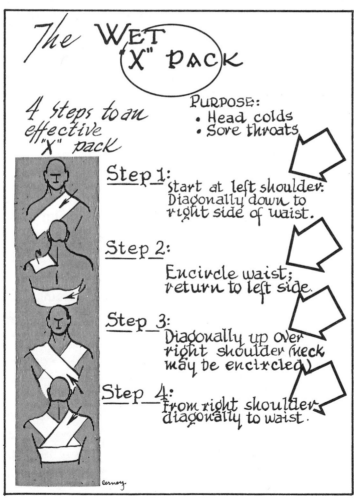

Figure 18

the sheet over the left shoulder. Working fast, bring it diagonally down to the right side of the waist, around the belt line, go to the left hip and diagonally up the chest to the right shoulder, diagonally down the back to the left hip and encircle the waist once more. Continue making "X'''s front and back until the end of the sheet. If any is left over, encircle the throat. Cover yourself with a blanket and sit in an easy chair to watch television or read. Remove as it warms. Dunk in cold water, squeeze dry and repeat. Repeat at least four times. On the fourth time around you will be very drowsy. Rub yourself down briskly and get into bed. Cover warmly and sleep.

At-a-Glance Information

Other Non-Health Problems
You Can Treat with the

WET "X" PACK

Neck: tonsillitis, colds, sore throats.

Note: always combine throat packs with the chest "X" pack to prevent congestion in the neck as a result of the changing circulatory apparatus,

Local: wounds, bruises, sprains, strains, ulcers, bites, stings, local infections and inflamation.

Grandpa used the "X" pack on me when I was a kid. In turn I've used it on my own five children and grandchildren as well. At first they protest. Then they start to look forward to it because it stops that head cold so fast. It gently lulls a person to sleep. As a sedative it can't be beat. Your head clears. You start breathing through your nose once more. Try it! One of the excellent fringe benefits from this therapy is that it's a preventive for future colds.

6. SUPPLEMENTARY TECHNIQUES

    A. Drink water and/or fruit juices copiously.
    B. Take vitamin A, C and D.
    C. Bed rest if you have the time and desire.

MOUTH

EFFECTIVE METHODS TO STOP
TOOTHACHE PAIN

A toothache is a neuralgic pain resulting from irritation, infection, or inflammation of the dental pulp. Remember that *a tooth is not bone*. It is made up of dentine encased in cement and covered with white enamel. Its roots are buried in the jaw. Blood vessels and nerves feed through its base. Quite often the local pain is NOT caused by a tooth. It may be a reflex pain originating somewhere else in the nervous system. In any case, from any cause, we all want relief from a toothache. To solve this problem let me tell you about Maxie T..

Maxie had pain in his lower jaw. He complained of excruciating agony. To verify my diagnosis of nerve involvement I referred Maxie to an oral surgeon who sent him back to me. "There's nothing I can do for him." That's when I started water therapy and it brought Maxie immediate results. Here's what we did:—

STEPS TO TAKE:

1. ICE RUB

Gently, with rotary motion, rub ice on the following points:—

a. *In front of the shoulder.*

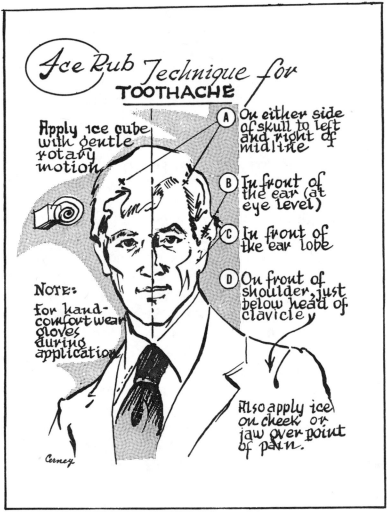

Figure 19

b. *In front of the ear*
c. *On the head*
   (see Figure 19).[4]

2. FINGER TIP PRESSURE TECHNIQUE
   (No Ice)

A. *Temple:* apply three finger tips on your temple on the

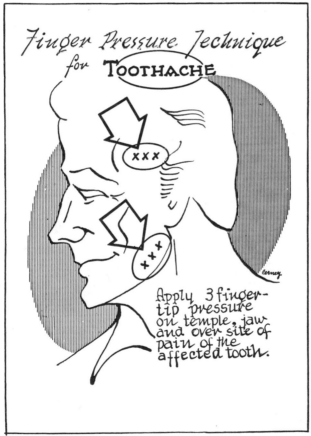

Figure 20

[4]Chinese acupuncture points. For further information on this excellent technique, see my book *Acupuncture Without Needles*, Parker Publishing Company, Inc., West Nyack, N.Y., 1974.

side of the toothache. Press for 10 seconds and release, then hold for one minute. Repeat at least five times.

B. *Jaw:* apply three finger tips on the jaw on the side of the hurt.

C. *Above and below the aching tooth*

**A Long Hidden Cerney-Secret
for Relief of Aching Teeth**

3. CAROTID ARTERY PRESSURE TECHNIQUE

Here is an amazing method that has worked for me—and my patients—for over a half century and will be worth a million to you in the future. Let's take the case of Chris K. as an example. Chris had a pain in his jaw that nobody could help. Anesthesia, oral sedatives, nothing stopped it. He identified the pain as feeling as though he was being stabbed in the face with an ice pick. He said it came and went. In between stabs was a persistent gnawing that drove him frantic. He was gaunt from loss of sleep and pain. He couldn't eat. Couldn't work. He could hardly move without pain shooting through his face. The surgeon suggested cutting nerves. The dentist was baffled because x-ray film and examination were totally negative. I couldn't find anything either until in checking his neck I found that the *carotid artery—on the side of the toothache—was pounding like a triphammer*! I took Chris' hand and placed three of his finger tips on that artery of his neck. I told him to press gently but firmly for a three count and then release; and then repeat the process three times and follow it with a cold wet towel around his neck. He was told to replace the cold therapy as the towel warmed. This went on for half an hour. When I returned to the treatment room he had a strange, almost bewildered, look of disbelief on his face. "Doc," he exclaimed, "it's gone!" And it was. And you can do the same for yourself.

My grandfather showed me this technique a long time ago and I've been using it ever since. Now I give it to you.

NOSE

HOW TO STOP THAT
NOSE BLEED
. . . FAST!

A *nosebleed* is any hemorrhage from the nostrils and it has many possible causes. The most common cause is that of "picking the nose." However, air conditioning, foreign bodies, a direct blow, sinus problems etc. are contributing problems. Nosebleeds may come as the result of systemic disease or be due to high blood pressure. From any cause, nosebleed may be successfully handled through water therapy. A good example of this was 69 year old Layne McG. Layne had hardening of the arteries. He also had high blood pressure. Every time he got excited his nose bled. This frightened him. He didn't realize that Nature was actually doing him a favor by relieving cranial pressure with a nosebleed, that it was a safety valve. Being frightened, he sought professional help as any sensible person should do. I explained the problem after making a complete physical examination and told him that he was in no danger, that what he *did* need was a method to control the bleeding in case the bleeding refused to stop. Here's the procedure suggested for Mr. McG. after his blood pressure was brought under control. You will find the method efficient and easy to do. What's best about it is that nosebleeds from any cause may be handled within moments in just this way.

STEPS TO TAKE:

1. CERNEY TECHNIQUE FOR NOSEBLEED

    A. *Pack 1" gauze* into nostril on side involved. DO NOT use cotton batting!

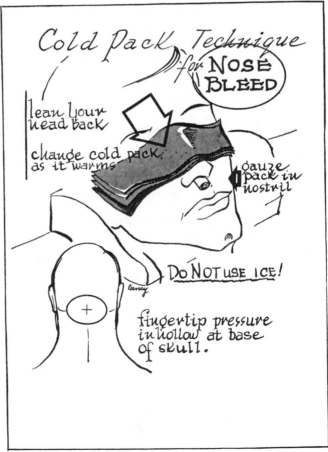

Figure 21

B. *Cold water foment* over bridge of nose (no ice!)

C. *Ice bag or cold pack* at nape of neck.

D. *Lean head back* while seated upright.

E. *Finger-tip pressure* in central hollow at the base of the skull.

Use both hands in applying rotary pressure with fingertip pressure in this area.

2. ICE CUBE OR COLD WATER TREADING TECHNIQUE

This method deals with reflexes on the feet. (See Figures 5 and 17.) Cold applications on the feet cause blood vessels in the body to constrict. This also applies to the blood vessels of the nose. Ice cube application to the little toe gets you your results. Simply massage the fatty ball of the toe and note how fast the bleeding stops. Cold water treading in the bathtub, lake, or stream acts in the same manner.

> *NOTE: In children, nosebleed may occur in measles, whooping cough, rheumatic fever, scarlet fever. It may also occur where there is a big absence of vitamin C in the diet. Use the same methods on the child's nosebleed as on the adult.*

HAY FEVER CURES
THROUGH THE MAGIC OF WATER THERAPY

Teenager Martha T. developed hay fever. In the springtime, pollens from oak, maple, birch, poplar, and elm trees started her itching. In the summer, pollens from Bermuda grass and timothy made this youngster sniffle, sneeze, and snort. Sending her out to the farm didn't help because wheat rust and corn pollen gave her fits and ragweed added insult to injury. First her nose started itching. Then the roof of her mouth itched. Itching and swelling began deep in her throat. Her eyes itched the most. They also watered furiously to rid themselves of the pollutants. She couldn't stand being in the light. Her nose ran like a drippy faucet. When I saw her for the first time, there was pain in her forehead as well as a queasy stomach which she reported. Her family said that she was irritable, refused to eat, and that they were up with her all night long. They just didn't know how to cope with the problem any more because nothing had proven effective. They admitted that Martha had had all the antihistamines and Neosynephrin nose drops, cortisone and ACTH "shots" and none of it had helped. They also said they couldn't afford the mountains or seashore as doctors had previously prescribed . . . and, was there anything—just anything—they could do at home to bring relief. I admitted it was a tough problem but possibly there WAS an answer. Perhaps the modern magic of natural healing with water therapy would do the trick. It did! After using the following water therapy, her hay fever hasn't bothered her since. She reported instant relief.

STEPS TO TAKE:

1. SINUS MASK (layers of dampened gauze, or nose filter)

The mask is worn over the nose and over the mouth during all pollen and dust-laden seasons. Martha wasn't too Gung-ho for the idea but she did it and was happy she did because results were immediate when the mask was used in conjunction with the—

2. COLD WET ABDOMINAL COMPRESS

Dunk folded toweling in cold water. Squeeze dry. Apply on the abdomen each morning and afternoon for an hour at a time. Re-apply as quickly as it warms.

3. BEDTIME COLD COMPRESSES

Martha was instructed on how to apply the bedtime compress as follows: As with the abdominal compress a folded towel is used. Saturate with cold water, squeeze dry and apply over the forehead and nose as well as the abdomen for one hour each night. Martha reported that they made her sleep. And it's true. When properly used, cold packs are the most wonderful sedative in the world.

4. SALT WATER RINSE OR LAVAGE

In one quart of cold water, dissolve one tablespoonful of common table salt. Cup the salty solution in your hands, Insert your nose into the liquid. Sniff it in. Pinch your nostrils together with thumb and index finger and throw your head back. Head forward, drain the solution. Repeat morning and night.

5. INTESTINAL LAVAGE (colonic or irrigation)

Apply twice daily for two weeks. (Review Figure 9.)

6. SUPPLEMENTARY INSTRUCTIONS

Take at least 100,000 units of Vitamin A per day for two weeks. Then 50,000 units per day for a month thereafter. Add Vitamin C ration. Eat fresh vegetables and fruit as your main staple. Lay off all sweets and pastries and avoid all coffee, tea, and soft drinks. Drink copiously of fresh fruit and vegetable juices. Eat less meat.

> *NOTE: When Martha came in for her last twice-a-year "checkup," she reported that very seldom now does she have reoccurrences of her allergies. I can't scientifically explain how the above procedures work when other specialists have failed. What I DO know is something that my grandfather said–"With water therapy you are always in the hands of God."*

HOW TO CONQUER YOUR
SINUS PROBLEMS

Inflamed sinuses are a common problem. They are becoming an even graver problem with air pollution lying like a blanket over the U.S.A. *Sinusitis* may come on suddenly or gradually. It may be caused by respiratory ailments (colds, influenza, bronchitis, etc.), changes of temperature, polyps in the nose, swollen turbinates, emotional upsets, allergies, and even abscesses in the jaw.

My former sparring partner, Jodie Farrar, had sinusitis. It came because he didn't keep his boxing guard up. A quick right to the beak and his deviated septum swelled immediately. It closed up his breathing apparatus. His sinuses filled and when this occured he had such fringe non-benefits as headache, nasal discharge and local pain. He felt awful all over, according to his statement. Every time his sinuses got involved he ran a fever (never over 103°F). There was dizziness, and general aches and pains. You could always tell which one of Jodie's sinuses was acting up because finger-tip pressure on it made him wince. Hit it with a gloved fist and he howled. Around his eyeball there was swelling. His upper teeth hurt. Sometimes he had pain at the back of his head, sometimes just behind his eyes or at the root of his nose. As a result, he became so depressed that it changed his personality. From an easy-going, happy-go-lucky guy he became progressively vicious. He started throwing dirty blows and he couldn't help it. Finally, realizing what was happening to Jodie, our trainer and manager, Willie D., put him on a hydrotherapy program that he'd picked up in Vienna during Jodie's overseas fights. This not only cleared up Jodie's problems but gave me a how-to-do-it sinus technique that I've used in my practice ever since. It was the same as I used on Martha T.'s hay fever.

STEPS TO TAKE:

1. NASAL SALT RINSE OR LAVAGE

Place a tablespoonful of table salt in one quart of water. Stir till salt dissolves. Scoop it up in both hands. As you lean over the wash basin, insert your nose. Breathe the solution up into your nose. Pinch nose shut. Throw head back. Lean forward. Release.

> *NOTE: In the beginning stages, your nose will be very tender inside. As the sensitivity diminishes, this will be your criterion of improvement. Alternate with a nasal irrigation.*

2. NOSE IRRIGATIONS

Utilizing a medicine dropper and a solution of salt water, bicarbonate of soda and boric acid, lean the head back so that the unaffected side of the nose is topside. With the irrigating container just an inch or so higher then the affected side of the nose, insert the catheter. With the mouth open so that you can breath freely through your mouth start the flow going. Irrigate each nostril with up to about five ounces of fluid. When finished DO NOT BLOW YOUR NOSE! Drip dry instead.

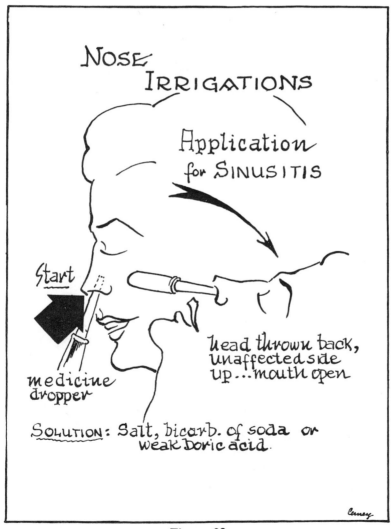

Figure 22

3. STEAM HUMIDIFICATION

Some folks get a great deal of relief for sinus problems by breathing steam. This is simple to accomplish at home. Just place a few drops of eucalyptus oil in a tea kettle after the water has been brought to a boil. Place the steaming kettle on the kitchen table. Sit down. Draw a turkish towel—or umbrella, or blanket—over your head. Breathe deeply inside your tent. This worked beautifully for Jodie Ferrara. He received instant relief.

4. PROPER NOSE-BLOWING HABITS

If you have sinus problems be cautioned about blowing your nose too hard or too often. Prefer to drip dry no matter what other people think. If you must blow, blow your nose gently on one side at a time. Keep your mouth closed while doing it.

5. GARGLE FREQUENTLY

Gargle salt solution (one tablespoonful per one quart of water) each morning and evening.

6. COLD PACKS OVER BRIDGE OF NOSE and an ice pack at the nape of the neck

7. SUPPLEMENTARY PROCEDURES

A. *Diet:* Eat lots of fresh vegetables and fruits. Take at least 100,000 units of Vitamin A per day. Add Vitamin C as well. No pastries or sugar, less meat.

B. *Bed rest* during the acute stage (if possible)

C. *Water and fruit juices* copiously.

These procedures have given relief to folks who have had no relief from any other kind of treatment. They're not complicated. Nothing hard to do, but in just a few moments you have relief. It's modern magic indeed!

SCALP

REVITALIZING YOUR SCALP
AND GROWING HAIR ONCE MORE

If your baldness occurs after an illness in which you have had a high fever, or had to take particular kinds of drugs, you can use water therapy to restore hair. If, however, you are from a family of bald heads don't expect water therapy to change the course of heredity. However, if you have a thin head of hair, it can become more luxuriant, more gleaming, more thick, through water treatment. *The secret lies in stimulating circulation to the scalp.* Hydrotherapy does just this and here are the—

STEPS TO TAKE:

1. HOT WET TURBAN FOLLOWED BY NEEDLE-POINT SPRAY

Fold a large turkish towel lengthwise in thirds. Saturate with hot water (115°F) and wrap the top of the head turban style. As your turban cools remove it, re-soak, wring dry, re-apply. Repeat for one hour. Follow this with a needle-point cold spray, or nozzle, as you stand in the bathtub. The spray head attached to your bathtub faucet should be adjusted to provide a sharp stinging impact. (Other nozzles and hoses are available at your hardware store.) Spray head should be at least 14 inches from your scalp and should not be so strong as to cause pain or discomfort. In water therapy we are concerned with the action and reaction to treatment and that's where the secret lies. Dry your head vigorously with a towel. *Do NOT use a hair dryer*! Keep the scalp cool to achieve best results. Repeat treatment on alternate evenings for a month (before bedtime). You will tingle. Your scalp will begin to feel warm. So will you. This method is excellent when most everything else fails. As a fringe benefit it should be noted that you can use this treatment for ear problems.

Mark V. had an interesting side effect from the hot-turban-cold-jet-spray routine. He dropped in to tell me that since using the jet spray technique his dandruff had completely disappeared. In this technique, no drugs or other care are necessary. Let Nature do what has to be done . . . notably restore circulation to the scalp . . . because Nature still remains the best doctor after all.

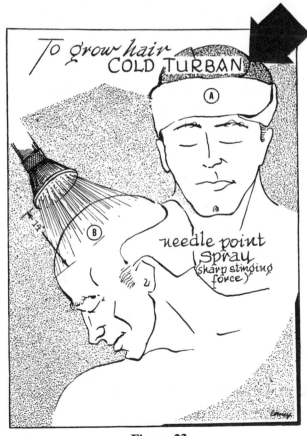

Figure 23

water

treatment

for the

NECK

---

chapter

2

Subjects covered:

Adenoids
Coughing
Goiter
Laryngitis
Pharyngitis
Swollen Throat ("Tonsillitis")
Torticollis ("Wry Neck")
"Whiplash" injury

ADENOIDS

A Child Finally Finds Relief
from a Neck Ailment

Although *adenoids* are no longer the problem they were years ago, the problem still makes itself painfully prominent at times, and water therapy is its best control. Adenoid inflammation is often associated with tonsillitis. The eustachian tubes may get involved and an earache result.

Little Maudie P. had this problem. Her adenoids swelled in winter and spring. Her throat swelled and she had to breathe through her open mouth. Her breath was terrible. She coughed and vomited and had a curiously strained look on her face. Maudie was one of those youngsters born with a high palate and dental problems. She constantly had an infection in her nose, her sinuses, tonsils and middle ear. Her neck was tender to touch and this kept on periodically with the family druggist on a yoyo between Chloromycetin and Aureomycin prescriptions. The drugs continued until the day we started water therapy. That's when Maudie's relief began. In all their simplicity here are the—

STEPS TO TAKE:

1. NASAL LAVAGE

Rinsing the nose is easily accomplished by cupping the hands, scooping up cold water (one tablespoonful salt in one quart of cold water), placing the nose down into the handcup of water and "breathing it in." Repeat four times. Because the coldness contracts tissues, Maudie's nose opened. She breathed through her nose for the first time in years. She repeated the process three times daily. The tissues toughened and remained "shrunken." In so doing, they became less susceptible to infection. She had fewer and fewer colds and no more swollen adenoids.

2. NECK WET PACK AND OR ICE COLLAR

Saturate a bath towel with cold water. Squeeze out the excess. Fold the towel lengthwise in fourths and wrap around the throat. Renew the wrap four or five times as it warms. Apply morning and night. An alternate to the wet pack is the ice collar. If a "collar" (rubber or plastic) is not available, simply use a sandwich bag filled with crushed ice and mould it around your throat.

3. FOOD CONTROL

Keep your diet light. Take nutritious fluids all day long (milk, milk shakes, fruit juices, vegetable juices, bouillon). I put little Maudie on this program and over the years I've watched her grow up. She's married now, has children of her own, and not once in those years did her adenoiditis return. What did it? The water cure. It worked for her. Why not for you?

HOW TO QUELL THAT IRRITATING COUGHING

Home folks are often confused about that forced expulsion of air from the lungs called "coughing." There are many forms of coughing. Each has a different cause and it's no wonder folks are confused. There's the bronchial cough, the asthmatic cough, the brassy cough, the hacking, the harsh, the hysterical, the short cough. Many serious ailments have coughing as a symptom. This is true of measles, pharyngitis, diphtheria, influenza and whooping cough. In the "common cold," coughing may accompany sneezing, "feeling bad," runny nose and a scratchy feeling in the throat. This hacking, non-productive cough is usually worse at night and interferes with sleep. But no matter what the cause there are particular water therapy procedures you can use to conquer your problem. Here are the—

STEPS TO TAKE:

1. COLD WET FOMENT

In the usual manner, saturate a large turkish towel with cold tap water. Fold lengthwise in fourths. Squeeze out excess water. While sitting in an easy chair, wrap the compress around your throat. Place a larger compress on your chest. Reapply as they become warm. Be certain that you cover the original area of irritation. This may take four or five applications. Leave the final foment in position and get into bed. Sleep between plastic sheets, or, utilize a little gimmick I developed to keep the bedclothing from getting saturated. What's the gimmick? Take a plastic garment bag that you get back from the cleaners with your clothing. Cut a hole at the top for your head and just enough out of the corners through which to push your arms. Sometime during the night you will awaken. Remove the plastic bag. Throw the compress on the floor. Towel yourself briskly and go back to sleep. Repeat the next day if coughing starts up.

I always used this method on my youngest daughter Kim whose sensitive nose starts her coughing every time she's exposed to pollen, dust and other noxious elements. In fact, I used this method on my entire family as well as on patients. If your cough is persistent here's the antidote—

PERSISTENT COUGHING THAT NEEDS EXTRA ATTENTION

STEPS TO TAKE:

1. ICE THERAPY

Rub an ice cube on the sides, back and front of your neck.

Keep the ice cube moving in a rotary motion. Do not use it if the skin blanches. Ice therapy is especially effective if followed by a cold wet foment. Treatment time for the ice cube "rub" is *until relieved*. Foments that follow should be repeated at least four times as they warm, or until such time as the cough disappears.

2. THROAT IRRIGATIONS

There are two approaches to the throat irrigation. One may be with the enema bag tube. The other may be by gargling. The solution used in either method is composed of one tablespoonful of table salt to one quart of water. Use warm water (105°F). Baking soda or boric acid may also be used. Attach the enema bag above head level. Lean forward with your face over the lavatory bowl. Insert the syringe into your widely opened mouth. Do not insert the irrigator tip past the first molars. The rush of water will do the job. Permit the water to flow steadily without harsh impact. Do not swallow any of the solution. Breathe through your nose. If breathing gets difficult, turn the irrigator off and rest. Start again. In gargling with the same solution merely throw your head back and let a column of air come up through the mouthful of fluid. Swish the water around in your mouth, expel and repeat.

HOW TO KNOCK OUT
WHOOPING COUGH

Prevention "shots" have reduced *pertussis* (whooping cough), but now and again youngsters "catch it anyhow." Here's the method to cope with it—

STEPS TO TAKE:

1. WARM FULL BATH (Review Figure 16)

Follow the warm bath with a quick, cold, stimulating shower.

2. COLD WET THROAT COMPRESS

Apply at bedtime, along with. . .

3. COLD WET ABDOMINAL COMPRESS

Apply firmly over the abdomen. Also give the child. . .

4. HOT LEMONADE

On the hour to prevent coughing, relieve spasms and clear the throat. *Note*: after the paroxysms have diminished, cut the lemonade down to every two hours.

WHAT TO DO, AND HOW, TO CONTROL YOUR GOITER
Via the Water Route

Mary R.—when she appeared in my office—presented not just a bulging neck but bulging eyeballs as well. She was frightening to look at as well as being an unusual medical marvel. Mary was 42 at the time. She was a hard-working, conscientious person and the health profile she presented was typically thyroid. Her hands trembled. Muscles in her arms twitched. Vomiting and diarrhea were daily occurrences. Her heart fluttered. She was anemic, had sugar in her urine and a high basal metabolism rate as well. She was a candidate for surgery but this she refused to have. She had earlier refused to take any more of the heavy medication that had been prescribed by previous physicians. Her thyroid kept enlarging. She had what is known as an *exophthalmic goiter* and certainly something had to be done. It was. Here's the natural healing procedure that Mary used and it changed the course of her life. The bulge retreated. Her shrewish personality sweetened. You won't believe it, but she got to looking so nice she decided to learn to dance at Arthur Murray's. The next thing I knew she was married. Modern magic at its best.

STEPS TO TAKE:

1. COLD WET PACKS

Fold a large towel lengthwise in the usual manner. Saturate with cold water and squeeze out the excess water. Wrap towel around your neck. Repeat as it warms. Treatment time is one hour. Two sessions daily.

2. CAROTID SINUS PRESSURE

This is truly your *magic button*. Find this "sinus" as fol-

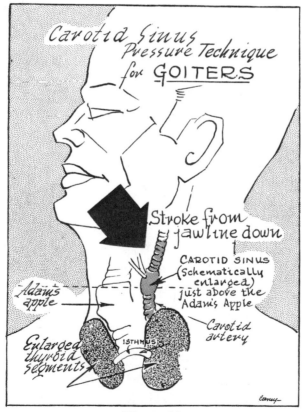

Figure 24

lows: Locate the top of your Adam's apple with your index finger tips. Then draw your fingers backward till you feel a pulse. "X" marks the spot. This is your key pressure point. Breathe deeply. Press both sides of the neck for a long five count. Exhale. Repeat again. Three repetitions are sufficient three times daily.

3. SUPPLEMENTARY PROCEDURES

A. *Sea Kelp* (high in iodine) may be obtained from your health food store or druggist.

B. Use only *iodized salt.*

C. Avoid all bean products, avoid cabbage. Both contain *cyanates,* a chemical known to produce goiters. Watch all drug labels and avoid those carrying such an ingredient.

HOW TO STOP
LARYNGITIS OVERNIGHT

There are various kinds of laryngitis. Each has a specific cause. Each has a specific treatment so that no one treatment is good for all. For example—a public speaker, or cheer leader, misusing or over-using his voice, develops a kind of catarrh of the throat. Soft tissues swell and the voice may be temporarily lost. When the epiglottis swells inside the throat, this is known as *edematous laryngitis.* A child with the croup has *spasmodic laryngitis.* The most common problem is catarrhal laryngitis and here is the antidote from the standpoint of water therapy:—

STEPS TO TAKE:

1. COLD WET FOMENT, around the throat, should remain in position until warm or dry. Change as it warms. Overlay with warm blanketing to maintain coldness.

2. SALT WATER GARGLE (weak, hot). Cupful on the hour.

3. WARM FULL BATH daily (Review Figure 16) followed by a quick cold shower.

4. WHAT TO AVOID. Tobacco, fumes, excesses in everything.

5. STEAM VAPORS (Review Figure 2) (with eucalyptus oil) may be used but are not of great value.

6. SALT WATER INTERNAL LAVAGE (one tablespoonful of table salt to one quart of warm water (100°F).

7. BACK, CHEST, NECK MUSCLE MASSAGE to release tensions.

8. DIETARY CONTROLS should consist of soft diet only, or, strictly liquids, until the throat is relieved. No milk! Ginger ale recommended.

9. COMPLETE REST means mind as well as body.

COUNTERING
PHARYNGITIS
With the "Tap Water Cure"

Refrigerator Repairman
Repairs Own Neck Problem

Physical or health problems often result from causes we least expect. It was that way with Jack D. He said he had a "lump" in his throat all the time and wanted to know if he had a tumor, or if there was a fish bone in his throat. He said his throat burned, that he was hoarse most of the time and found it difficult to swallow. Sometimes his neck swelled, got tender and stiff. Sometimes he had chills and fever, and his nose ran. He kept rubbing his runny nose on the back of his hand during the entire examination. Everything in his examination proved negative including his throat so I questioned him about his occupation. Jack was a refrigerator repairman. He said there wasn't anything about his job that could bother him except when he put charges of Freon in refrigeration equipment. That's when his eyes lit up. He'd made his own diagnosis. Suddenly he was aware that when gas escaped the lump in his throat came back. That's when he had trouble with his throat. Whether your pharyngitis is from foreign irritants, such as gas or chemicals, or whether it is from bacteria, you can handle it adeptly with the following home therapy—

STEPS TO TAKE:

1. AVOID ALL AGGRAVANTS

Seek out, identify, and eliminate all chemical, thermal or other aggravations that bring on such an "attack" of pharyngitis. Simply stay away from all offending agents.

2. HOT/COLD COMPRESSES

To get the most out of this treatment place the *COLD pack on the back of the neck* and *HOT on the front.* Change the cold pack as it warms. Re-saturate with cold water, squeeze out the excess, and re-saturate with cold water, Repeat three times daily for 30 to 60 minutes per treatment.

3. COLD FOOT TUB BATH

By this method you activate reflexes beneficial to pharyngitis. Fill a bucket with cold water. Insert feet for three minutes. Remove, rub briskly with coarse toweling and don warm footgear. Repeat process twice daily.

4. DIETARY CONTROLS

In pharyngitis food control is vital. Eat only soft foods during the acute stage (soup). Drink NO TEA, COFFEE or COLA DRINKS, or MILK. Drink ginger ale. Add Vitamin A (100,000 units per day), Vitamins D and C to your diet.

HOW TO HANDLE THAT
SWOLLEN THROAT
(Tonsillitis)

Tiny Tot's Tonsillitis
Stopped by Water Treatment

A swollen throat is no fun. When tonsillitis occurs, swelling may be inside that throat as well as out and a whole train of uncomfortable symptoms follows. The first time I saw Nancy D. was backstage before a dancing-school recital. My daughters, Lee and Pat, were in it too. Nancy was a cute youngster and I became interested in her health when I saw her mother stuffing her with aspirin. Like any concerned backstage parent I enquired about Nancy and was informed that she was having chills, fever, and had a headache, that she had big bumps in her neck and that her body ached so badly that the mother didn't let her go to school that day. She said Nancy was coughing constantly and the more she coughed, the stiffer her neck became, and if aspirin didn't work she was going to have to take her home, dance revue or no dance revue. She admitted it was an idiotic thing even to have the child out of bed but any parent with a child in dancing school knows just how much youngsters look forward to this great occasion. She asked spontaneously if I would look at Nancy. I did. The procedures I recommended got Nancy through the revue. Therapy that followed eliminated the tonsillitis. She's grown up now and I take care of her children and they too are going to be in a dancing revue soon . . . without acute tonsilitis.

Note: In acute catarrhal type of tonsillitis the tonsils get red, swollen, enlarged. The walls around them get angry and the throat gets sore even as the nose and voice box become involved. In the acute follicular type of tonsillitis, crypts or pits begin to show in the swollen tonsil. These caves may fill with pus and debris. Fever and chills may follow. There's discomfort on swallowing. The entire body feels "bad all over." This is due to the fact that tonsillitis, even though it appears to be a local problem, spreads toxic waste through the entire body.

STEPS TO TAKE:

1. COLD PACKS ON THROAT TWICE DAILY

Fold a turkish towel lengthwise to a width that will fit the throat. Saturate with cold water. Squeeze. Encircle the throat. Go about your regular business. As soon as it warms, remove, re-saturate, wring dry and re-apply. Repeat as often as desired. This is wonderfully relaxing before bed time and induces sleep.

2. COLD HIP SITZ BATH (Review Figure 12)

3. DIETARY CONTROLS

A. Vitamins A,C,D

B. Soft foods ONLY (soups)

C. NO MILK! (ginger ale approved) (Also fruit and vegetable juices.)

4. MASSAGE

Relax all muscles of the chest, neck and back. Do it gently but well.

5. REST IN BED

6. HOT FULL BATHS

Quick relief from discomfort may come through hot eliminative and sedative baths. That general soreness and tired feeling are eliminated. Treatment time: 15 minutes. Follow with a quick cold shower and friction rub. Maintain water in tub at 102°F.

7. COLD WATER GARGLES

Gargling every half hour reduces the redness and swelling. DO NOT USE HOT medicated gargles.! You are only adding more fire to fire and slowing up the processes of healing.

8. COLD ENEMA OR COLONIC IRRIGATION DAILY. (See Figure 9)

WHAT TO DO ABOUT
TORTICOLLIS
(Wry Neck")

Marjorie C. was in an automobile accident. As a result of all the crazy pain she was going through she ran from doctor to doctor. The doctors pronounced her problem as *torticollis* and told her how it could be handled. She didn't listen. The problem got worse. Muscles on the side of her neck were in constant spasm. Her head pulled toward her left shoulder with her chin pointed to the right until it was impossible for her to look straight ahead.

When I first saw Marjorie she was gaunt. Her face was lined. She hadn't eaten in days. She was exhausted, wild-eyed, shrill, tearful, sarcastic, and totally un-nice. We went through an ordeal examining her but the examination was fruitful. X-ray film of her neck revealed the first cervical vertebra to be subluxated (out of joint) from its normal alignment. Her head was actually off its base. The neck muscles, in spasm, made the problem worse. Here's how she got relief—

STEPS TO TAKE:

1. MASSAGE

Massage neck, chest, and shoulders mildly with the initial approach to this problem. Follow with—

2. COLD COMPRESSES

Apply compresses on the upper back and neck (saturated cold toweling). Treat twice daily for two weeks investing an hour per treatment time. Note the gradual relaxation of muscles and this is the secret of what you're after.

3. PRESSURE POINT THERAPY

Place your thumbs in the hollow at the base of your skull. It will be very painful. Maintain pressure or make rotary motion with the thumb until the discomfort subsides. (One side of the hollow is usually more tender so keep at it) Now check the back of your shoulders. Note the knots of tension. Insert your index finger tip, like a claw, into each "ouch" area that you locate. Hold the pressure until you feel the muscle wiggle and release beneath your finger tip.

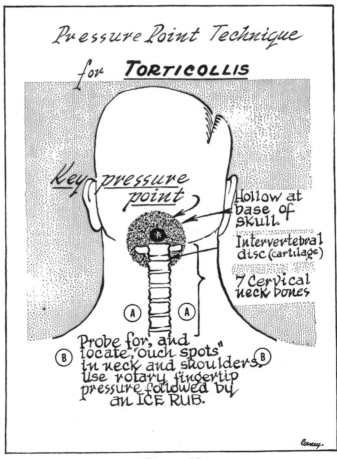

Figure 25

4. ICE RUB

Ice procedures may begin as soon as muscle relaxation begins. You, or a friend, can do this simply by rubbing an ice cube from ear to ear—with rotary motions—along the base of the skull. *Pinpoint the "ouch" areas. Mark them! They are the key to your problem!* Be gentle but firm in contact. At first each "ouch" zone will hurt on pressure. Slowly it will become insensitive as improvement takes place.

5. RELAXING FULL TUB BATH (Review Figure 16)

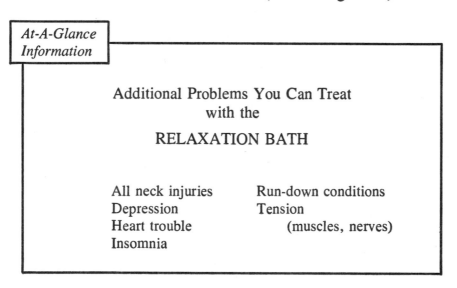

At-A-Glance Information

Additional Problems You Can Treat
with the

RELAXATION BATH

All neck injuries   Run-down conditions
Depression   Tension
Heart trouble   (muscles, nerves)
Insomnia

WHIPLASH INJURY
and How to Relieve Its Agonies

One of the growing problems in the U.S.A. is neck injury due to rear-end collisions. In this "accident" the head is suddenly and forcefully whipped back and then forward. Ligaments are stretched. Muscles, nerves, and bones of the neck become immediately involved. Some are stretched. Some torn. The sympathetic nervous system is also involved. As a result a lot of bizarre symptoms occur. Some of these appear to be totally unrelated to the accident and too often the person is accused of malingering. Doctors worth their salt are beginning to realize how inadequate has been their own understanding of this dangerous problem. One of the technical handles given to "whiplash injury" is *cervico-myofascitis*.

The Whiplash Injury of a News Photographer and How It Was Handled

Harvy DeM. was one of many piled up on a foggy, Dayton super highway en route to Cincinnati, Ohio. One automobile hit the other in a chain reaction. Harvey is a news photographer.

When I first saw Harvey he was no longer his exuberant self. His head was pulled over to the left side. His neck was rigid as well as swollen. Shoulder and back muscles were in violent spasm so that he couldn't turn his head or his body. He was mentally dull and complained of the desire to fall to one side, that he was totally washed out, had blackouts, and at times didn't know exactly where he was. And that's the way it was before he even started hitting the bottle to find relief. He said he "felt heavy," that his arms were like lead and that his hands and feet were tingly, cold and numb.

I was interested to note the change in personality that had taken place. He was no longer the debonair, outgoing sophisticate. He had become irritable, morose, inverted, short of breath, complained of nausea and vomiting and that his low back hurt, that he had pain between his shoulder blades and was constantly sweating.

As if this wasn't enough he couldn't remember anything. He couldn't concentrate. In fact, he hardly even remembered the accident. Anxious one minute, totally depressed the next. His heart beat like a triphammer and his eyes fought bright light. He couldn't sleep. He was going through that unique kind of hell that whiplash injury patients go through. He went from doctor to doctor seeking relief. Some told him all these symptoms didn't exist. It was all in his mind, that he was goofing off, looking to make a big kill in an insurance payoff. Neurosurgeons put him through the mill and it was like that—hospital after hospital with physicals, x-ray investigations, tests etc., etc. Finally his brother brought him in to see me. I also put him through the mill. It was *cervico-myofascitis* all right . . . a Grade-A whiplash injury with all its bizarre signs and symptoms showing. After some x-raying and medical manipulation of neck vertebrae, the following program was given him. He followed it religiously. Within a week's time he was back on the job. His insurance representative came in and asked, "What in the world did you do in a week's time that the big specialists and hospitals didn't accomplish in all these months of exhaustive and expensive investigation?" Well here's the program we followed:—

STEPS TO TAKE:

1. *See your bone manipulator first* (Osteopath, Chiropractor etc.) Let him check you out. Follow with the following routine:—

2. ICE THERAPY

Apply ice immediately to the back of the neck and muscles of the shoulders. Do this immediately after an accident. Fill a plastic bag with crushed ice. Lean back into an easy chair with the ice bag at the back of your neck. This position may be maintained for at least 30 to 60 minutes.

3. FULL RELAXATION BATH (Review Figure 16)

Apply this bath daily for its sedative and relaxant capabilities. Follow bath with a gentle massage and go to bed.

4. MASSAGE

To be applied daily on neck, shoulder and chest muscles. Follow with:—

5. COLD COMPRESSES

To the back, neck and shoulders for an hour each day.

water

treatment

for the

SHOULDER

---

chapter

3

Subjects covered:

Arthritis
Bursitis

BREAKING THE INFLAMMATION BARRIER
IN ARTHRITIS

For years I was an athletic trainer (see my textbooks[1]) and team doctor. I saw amateurs and professionals come and go. Injuries were numerous. However, aches and pains, which seemed to have no specific origin, often appeared. One of them was *arthritis*.

In studying the problem of arthritis—in and out of athletics—I began to realize that the word itself (*arthro-joint; itis*-inflammation) covered a multitude of sins. It's an easy word to say when one doesn't honestly know the cause. It sounds like something terrible and the average person knows little about it. Therefore, to help you make just a little more sense out of your shoulder aches remember that there are six (6) different kinds of arthritis. Some have to do with infections, some with disease, some with aging and deterioration, some with disturbed metabolism, as gout, some with glandular disturbances. It's all very complicated and confusing but remember the word break down—*arthro*-joint; *itis*-inflammation.

Inflammation means heat. So rather then add local heat to an already existing fire, the objective is to quell it to bring relief. For this prupose, cold hydrotherapy is most advantageous. The modern magic of natural healing through water therapy is the treatment of choice where shoulder problems are concerned.

It is true that heat *seems* to relieve shoulder or other joint pain. This, however, is strictly temporary. The heat may be in

---

[1] Cerney, J.V. *Care of Athletic Injuries*, C.C. Thomas Publishing Co. Springfield, Ill., 1963.

Cerney, J.V. *Athletic Taping Techniques*, Parker Publishing Company, Inc. West Nyack, N.Y., 1972.

the form of a heating pad, infrared lamp, shortwave machine, ultrasonic, or a hot shower or water bottle; and in this case I'm against them all. The only hot application in shoulder problems is the moist heat of a flaxseed poultice. (See Figure 26.)

> An exception to this is the person with rheumatoid arthritis who complains of early morning stiffness. Pain and stiffness decrease with activity as the day goes along. A full hot bath, immediately upon rising in the morning, will help start the day *but exercising the joint must follow immediately!*

For the most part, shoulder "arthritis" is a problem of *fibromyositis* or *myositis* (muscle inflammation) with pain, tenderness, and stiffness as the end result. The muscles and ligaments are involved. This may come without warning. This same myositic pain is what the doctors once called "rheumatism." When this same pain goes down the back it is called "lumbago." In the legs, it's called "charley horse" and in the neck it's called "torticollis." Therefore, in quelling this "itis," or heat, stick to cold water therapy. The following tells you how:—

STEPS TO TAKE:

1. COLD WET COMPRESSES (Review Figure 1). Reapply the packs as they warm.

2. CONTRAST BATHS may take place in the shower, or, with compresses. *Time of treatment:* two minutes in hot, one minute in cold. Repeat process five times alternately hot and cold.

3. TRACTION FOLLOWED BY MASSAGE of the neck, shoulders, and back. Stretch muscles by suspending by one hand from an overhead pipe or bar with the feet off the ground. Turn slowly left and right. This is one of the exercises used by baseball pitchers.

4. DIETARY CONTROLS. Cut down on ALL meats, pas-

tries and sugars. Stick to fresh vegetables and fruits. Drink plenty of vegetable and fruit juices. Take cod liver oil in tomato juice (tablespoonful daily).

5. COLONIC IRRIGATION (Review Figure 9) to cleanse the bowels. Evenings. Add one teaspoonful of salt to one quart of tepid water.

6. SLING OR FLEXIBLE CAST (adhesive tape bandage) may be used until shoulder muscle spasm subsides and/or the pain diminishes.

SHOULDER BURSITIS
and What to Do to Feel Better Faster

We are born with many bursa sacs. Some we develop. All of them have a duty. Their job is to cushion, protect, and lubricate friction and pressure areas. They may be just under the skin or down deep and communicate with a joint. Anything that irritates a bursa causes it to become inflamed. That's how its name developed:—*bursa* plus *itis* (inflammation) = bursitis. It may occur on a big toe joint from the rubbing of a shoe. A crapshooter may get it on his knees. People who sit too much may get it where they sit down. Acute bursitis may follow injury or unusual exercise. It may come with infection. By any route, the bursa sac fills with fluid, swells, gets extremely tender and limits function of the person who has it. Cap K. had bursitis in his shoulder from pitching soft ball. Mabel D. had it in her feet from wearing too narrow shoes. Each was given the following kind of therapy.

STEPS TO TAKE:

1. REMOVE THE CAUSE

2. ICE THERAPY

Rub the area involved with ice until it begins to ache. Do it gently. Follow each application of ice with the warm palm of your hand. Wait until the skin of the shoulder warms under your hand. Re-apply the ice. Alternate for at least four repetitions. Follow in the evening with—

3. COLD COMPRESSES

Cold compresses may be applied over or around all joints but the elbow. NOTE: *use no ice on the elbow!* (as in "Tennis Elbow") Toweling or other cloth—four thicknesses—is laid on the offended area. Permit it to become warm. Then back to the cold water, wring dry and re-apply. Repeat at least a half dozen times before bedtime. Then cover up warmly or don warm pajamas, trousers, sweater, shoes, whatever to keep the part warm as reaction from cold therapy sets in.

water

treatment

for the

UPPER

EXTREMITIES

---

chapter

4

Subjects covered:

Burns
Cold Hands
Neuralgia
Rheumatism

HOW TO GIVE YOURSELF FAST RELIEF
FROM BURNS

Fishing Guide Heals
Burns with Ice Water

Burns don't always end in permanent destruction of human tissue. How deep the burn extends is dependent on the intensity and duration of the exposure to the source of the heat, and the treatment that follows. Burns may result from thermal, electrical, chemical, radioactive causes, or even from friction. Gases may cause burns. Severe burns may produce shock and other complications. If treated promptly and properly with the magic of water therapy, complications to burns may be alleviated.

A good case on this score was Sam. Sam was not yet as old as the forest, but truly old and ages wise. He was an Ojibway. Full-blooded. From the past he brought—as did my grandfather from Europe—a wealth of Indian lore that brought me rudely awake to the fact that our stainless-steel today is very little newer than yesterday. This came to my attention when Sam, acting as guide on a fishing expedition, was scalded with boiling coffee.

We'd turned in for the night. The Canadian sun had set and when the fish stories got further apart we crawled into our sleeping bags. As usual Sam slept under the canoe. It acted as a lean-to and caught the heat from the nearby fire banked for the night. Balanced on supportive stones, and kept near the boiling stage, was the coffee pot, a big one.

Sometime during the night, we were rousted up by a family of overly hungry black bears tearing at our gear. They just wouldn't run. Sam reached for the coffee pot to give them a warm welcome. It toppled and spilled over his hands and arms.

While he shouted instructions to the rest of us, he ran down to the ice cold lake and thrust his hands and arms in.

Hours later, by the dawn's early light, I examined his extremities. No blisters! I didn't believe it! No redness! No loss of function! It was a little miracle due to hydrotherapy know-how. Nature's own remedy, a water cure that I saw happen in front of my own eyes!

STEPS TO TAKE:

1. CLEANSE BURNED AREAS IMMEDIATELY

Wash with soap and salt water. Follow with Step 2.

2. ICE WATER IMMERSION

Plunge the involved areas immediately into ice water. Keep inundated for at least 20 minutes or until the pain subsides. Remove. DO NOT DRY! Go to the next Step. If blisters are present DO NOT BREAK BLISTERS! Ice care for more extensive burns of the body is accomplished by immersing the entire body and maintaining cold temperature with ice cubes. *Time:* 20 minutes or until the pain stops.

3. WET DRESSING

Maintain all wet dressings for at least 24 hours. Soak toweling with salt solution. Follow this with a dry sterile gauze dressing. DO NOT APPLY PETROLEUM JELLY or other ointments. Grease merely houses secondary infections, should a blister break.

4. SALT SUPPLEMENTATION TO DIET

Sodium Chloride (salt) must be ingested internally to make up for loss that occurs in burns.

HOW TO GET COLD HANDS
WARM AGAIN

Water Treading for
Cold Hands

One of the most fascinating capabilities of the human body is that of the reflex action. A reflex is an action at one point that stimulates a reaction somewhere else. For example, tap the knee and the foot jerks. Shine a bright light in the eye and the pupil contracts. One of the most active of these reflexes is the one that controls the hands by treating the feet, back or neck. The person who has cold hands not only knows the discomfort cold hands bring, but wants a way to alleviate the problem. There *is* a way. It's simple. (Review Figure 5). Fill your bathtub with cold water as high as the calf of your leg. Get in. Walk back and forth. Lift your feet. This is called "water treading" and should be done each morning and night for five minutes per session. Get out. Rub feet briskly with a coarse towel, get stockings and shoes on and go about your duties. Variations on this are:—(a) *walking in the dewy grass barefooted each morning* (b) *spraying the feet* with cold water while sitting on the bathtub rim, (c) *cold hip sitz bath* (10 minutes) each evening before bedtime (Review Figure 12), (d) *ice pack on the back of the neck.*

WHAT TO DO ABOUT STOPPING
NEURALGIC PAIN

STEPS TO TAKE:

1. ICE THERAPY

Follow the course of the pain, with your fingertips, from shoulder to fingers. Mark the course with a soft pencil. Note that the pain follows a channel. Follow this channel with an ice cube. Make slow rotary motions along the entire course. After each excursion, run the warm palm of your hand, or a hot towel, down the same route. Then repeat the process twice again. At no time permit the skin to become blanched!

VICTORY OVER
RHEUMATISM

The pain and discomfort of rheumatism usually come on suddenly. There's no warning, no precursors, just pain aggravated by activity. The pain may be over a larger area or it may be localized to one "ouch" spot. Rheumatism has a way of following infections or some kind of poison that has been ingested into the body. It may come in the wake of a direct blow or exposure to dampness and cold. The muscles and fibers around the muscles don't like this kind of influence and they cry out in the form of aching or pain. Sometimes the muscles quiver or jump. Lindsey McD. got his "rheumatiz" working around a fishing dock on Kentucky's Cumberland Lake. Constant exposure to wind, rain and dampness finally got him to aching. While he was admiring the white bass I'd brought in, he told me about his problem. I asked him what he was doing for it. He showed me a copper band around his wrist and complained that "It warn't much good." I told him about Epsom salts baths and he said—"Well that probably ain't much good neither." So the next time I was down at Cumberland fishing, I asked him about his "rheumatiz." He showed me his wrist, The copper band was gone. He grinned a mouthful of toothlessness and said—"Ain't had a bit of trouble since I started using them Epsom salts bath you told me about. My wife likes them baths too. Says I even smell better."

STEPS TO TAKE:

1. EPSOM SALTS BATH

Mix Epsom salts slowly into hot water (120°F) in your bathtub. Purpose? Get rid of poisonous waste in the body. Salts accomplish this by dissolving urates and neutralizing toxins in the blood stream and body tissues. As an added plus, the treatment softens the skin. The technique is very important. Here's how to do it:—

Run approximately one inch of water into the bathtub. Mix in one pound of Epsom salts. Mix well. Now sit in the tub. Turn the water on slowly. While the tub is collecting another inch of water start rubbing yourself all over with a salt-water-saturated soft towel. When the water is up the second inch add another pound of Epsom salts. Continue the rub. At three inches, add another pound of salts. Continue the rub from head to foot. Here, now, is the big secret to this treatment:—

When sweat breaks out on your forehead QUIT! The treatment is terminated! Stand up. Take a quick cold shower. Rub down briskly with a dry coarse towel. Treatment time is approximately 12 to 15 minutes. Use this procedure only twice weekly. (Absolutely no more often!)

NOTE: If you would enjoy your bath by nose as well as by body add pine powder. This will give you a delightfully pungent bath and a gently soft skin.

At-a-Glance Information

Additional Problems You May
Treat with:
EPSOM SALTS BATHS

Rheumatism, sciatica, arthritis, lumbago, neuritis, colds and catarrh.

Problems You Should NOT Treat:

Do NOT take Epsom salts baths if you have a heart problem of any kind!

water
treatment
for the
CHEST

---

chapter
5

Subjects covered:

Asthma
Breath (shortness of)
Bronchitis
Heart
Pleurisy
Pneumonia
"Shingles"

ASTHMA
. . . and an Effective Way to
Breathe Easier Again

When an allergy affects any part of the breathing apparatus, strange sounds develop in the neck and chest. This inflammatory involvement is called *asthma*. It may be caused by dust, pollen, food, gases, bacteria, or chemical fumes. Damp and cold weather may aggravate it. It may be inherited. Asthma may have its inception in something as simple as an irritated nasal membrane or in something as complicated as an abnormality in the diaphragm. Your physician is the one to determine this matter. Climate, gout, sexual intercourse, etc. may bring on an "attack."

When Jeannie R. had asthma for the first time she thought it was nothing more then a tummy ache because she experienced gas in her abdomen. Along with tummy ache she got chilly, and then depressed. Her chest felt full. Her nose and throat itched. Her breathing became more and more difficult. Coughing ended with expectoration or spitting up. The incessant coughing also ended her job as a telephone company operator. What was further significant about Jeannie's case was that between "attacks" she had absolutely no symptoms! When the "attacks" occurred closer together, I saw her for the first time. The following program was set up for her. She responded exceedingly well and the telephone company hired her back.

STEPS TO TAKE:

1. DETERMINE THE CAUSE

2. LOCAL HOT "X" PACK (Review Figure 18)

     Place hot pack over the chest and thoracic (back) vertebrae

when asthma comes on at night. Alternate with cold compresses once weekly over the same area of the back. *Treatment time:* 30 minutes for both "X" packs and compress.

3. MUSCLE MASSAGE

Loosen all muscles of the neck, back, and shoulders, as well as the chest. Do this three times weekly. Get all muscles into a relaxed state. Work out the "knots." Follow this with—

4. FRICTION RUB

The million dollar "Friction Rub" is a key to "cures" and the maintenance as well as improvement of health!

The Dr. Monod Glove-Rub and How It Works

The normal instinct is to rub something that hurts. Nature tells us instinctively what to do. So why not take advantage of our instincts to improve and maintain our health? Why not utilize the magic of a normal physiological phenomenon by "rubbing what hurts"—or even rubbing areas around it? Why not develop a million-dollar friction rub that—in three or four minutes each day—can make you "feel like a million again!"

Can this be done? It can!

Gustave Monod, many years ago, in Paris, developed a system of skin rubs. After a full bath (120°F), he advocated goat skin gloves because of the effective friction they provided. What he found was that friction on the skin is of great importance to health, that it not only keeps the skin clean, but that three or four minutes daily devoted to improving circulation moved the vital properties of metabolism to areas of need. Muscles were given new tone, the nervous system quieted down, the mind became clearer, the stomach and bowels became less tender, digestion improved, intestinal and urinary secretions were regulated, and as all these functions improved, the very diseases sponsored by their weakness began to disappear!

Asthma, anemia, dyspepsia, constipation, nephritis, excessive fat, all are alleviated through the process of stimulating and returning the body to normal physiological processes once more. All through a "friction rub."

Sounds fantastic? It's not. It's just plain fact! It's just plain taking advantage of the very tools God gave us in the first place. It's merely stepping up physiological action through friction on our body. Use it! It's the very stepper-upper you may have been looking for.

Gustave Monod did it with gloves. He produced a feeling of well-being through friction rubbing. But so did the Swedes. In Old Europe, the *"Swedish Salt Glow"* is the epitome of the external bath and friction rub.

Swedish Salt Glow Helps Restore Health and Beauty

The *"Swedish Salt Glow"* is the process of taking a full hot bath until perspiration breaks out on the forehead, standing up, rubbing the skin briskly with dry table salt until the body is glowing pink, taking a quick cold shower, rubbing down with a coarse towel and jumping into bed. Sleep comes on quickly, so beautifully. The next morning you feel like a million. Friction rub! It prepares mind and body to fight off anything. It builds body resistance. It helps you get rid of fat. Use friction rubs and you help yourself to health! The friction rubs are my first suggestion for the asthmatic patient.

5. PRESSURE POINT CONTROL

Of great value in asthma. In all asthmatics there are little areas or "bumps" that can be felt on the chest. Go ahead! Probe your own chest. Get deep into the tissues without being rough. Some of these nodules will be so tender they can hardly be touched. It is very possible you have noticed these "ouch spots" in the past, wondered about them and promptly forgot them. Well don't forget them again. They are your health triggers. Use them! Seek them out and treat them with a vibrating or rotary pressure of the fingertip. In asthma, be more concerned with "ouch spots" *high* on the chest wall rather then with those on the rib cage below. (When we come to heart treatment you will see why.)

6. DIETARY CONTROLS

What you eat may not be the source of allergy causing asthma but *how much* you eat and WHEN you eat it may be the cause. My instructions to Jeannie R. were simple: "NO HEAVY MEALS AT ANY TIME! NO EVENING MEALS at any time. No sweets or gas-forming foods such as beans, cabbage, pastries, etc. "As a result of the above regimen Jeannie hasn't had one leave of absence from her job since.

FOR THE CHRONIC ASTHMATIC

STEPS TO TAKE:

1. WARM FULL BATH (98°F-Review Figure 16) ten minutes each evening, followed by—

2. HOT PACK ON ABDOMEN all night or until asleep.

3. COLD SHOWER EACH MORNING upon awakening

4. FOR EMERGENCY ATTACKS:
   A. *Hot foot or hand* (or both) *baths* with
   B. *Ice packs or cold compresses* on the head and back of neck.
   C. *Hot packs over the chest* followed by a brisk rubbing of the skin with cold water.

5. HOT ENEMA or colonic irrigation repeated every 30 minutes or until the asthmatic spasms stop.

6. HALF HIP-SITZ BATH (Review Figure 12) (80°-85°F) ten minutes, with cold affusions (pouring) and brisk rubbing of

cold water on the back and neck. If you have someone to rub your back and neck, rub your own chest simultaneously for more effective results.

7. RUSSIAN BATH (steam cabinet) for 20 minutes AFTER the initial sweat breaks out on the forehead. Older folks should remain in the cabinet only ten minutes. Follow all Russian baths with a cold shower. *Note:* everyone with heart problems should avoid this procedure.

HOW TO RELIEVE
SHORTNESS OF BREATH

STEPS TO TAKE:

Immerse hands and arms into hot water (110°-120°F) and rub them briskly. This may also be done with a watering can or spray in the bathtub. Follow this with a brisk rubbing of the dry arms and hands. This is of particular value in bronchitis, pneumonia, or tuberculosis which contribute to the shortness of breath. Apply cold compresses on the chest and lay back. Go to sleep.

IN EMERGENCY . . . WHEN BREATHING
APPEARS TO HAVE STOPPED

Apply cold water (ablution) to the back of the neck and head. Rub vigorously. Grasp the tip of the fifth finger. Whirl it around as if winding a handle. Then do the other hand. Repeat the same process on the third finger of each hand. This is an Oriental emergency measure that I pass on to you. The technique comes from Japanese *Shiatsu.*

HOW TO OVERCOME
BRONCHITIS

How a Factory Worker
Solved His Problem

Bronchitis is any inflammation of the bronchial mucous membrane and trachea. This inflammation may be caused by bacterial disease, cold, dust, or the inhalation of noxious gases. In its beginning stages, bronchitis has little more then a cough as a symptom. It's a dry, rough cough. The cough comes in spasms. As the mucous membrane dries out, the chest begins to feel uncomfortable. There's pain and a feeling of fullness in the chest. Breathing may get a little difficult.

John M. had all this and something added. He went on to chest pain that felt raw inside. When he coughed, stabbing pains wracked his chest. He had fever of 103°F and headaches. After exertion, he could scarcely breathe. As far as John's problem was concerned, it was *chronic bronchitis* and the treatment was different from that for *acute* bronchitis. Treatment was as follows. Within a month he was back to his old self again. He rejoined his buddies in scuba and deep sea diving since he could use his lungs again.

STEPS TO TAKE:

HOW TO TREAT
CHRONIC BRONCHITIS

1. HOT MUSTARD FOOT BATH (110°F) 20 minutes. Place one tablespoonful of powdered mustard in bucket of hot water.

2. MILD MUSTARD PLASTER on the chest. (See Figure 26).

"Plasters" or Poultices and How to Make Them

"Plasters" are yet another form of applying local heat. Mustard, flaxseed, or even mud have been used for centuries for the purpose of relieving local pain through retaining heat over an extended period of time. Flaxseed does this efficiently. Mustard, on the other hand, is a counter-irritant. It gets the skin red over the affected area and as this action takes place, a reflex occurs in the body. Local nerve ends are dulled and the pain is thus relieved. Mustard releases a highly volatile oil that creates this reaction. Flaxseed releases nothing but the heat it has absorbed in preparation.

Here's the Recipe

Mustard plasters are one part mustard mixed with six parts of baking flour (12 parts of flour for children). Add warm water to make a paste. Place doughy mess on a piece of cloth. Spread a quarter-inch thickness to a size large enough to cover the offended area to be treated. Bring the edges of the cloth up on top so that there will be no leakage of the contents. Cover with a plastic sheet or damp towel. Overlay with a hot water bottle. Do not leave "plaster" on too long. Blistering will occur.

Bronchitis is divided roughly into acute and chronic classifications. This is not to make everything more complex but to simplify the fact that the treatment for each is somewhat different. For example, people with *acute bronchitis should have MOIST air to breath!* The person with *chronic bronchitis should breathe DRY air*. If you have acute bronchitis, here's the way to handle it:—

3. HOT "X" PACK to be applied on the neck and chest. (Review Figure 18.) Change on the half hour or as it warms and

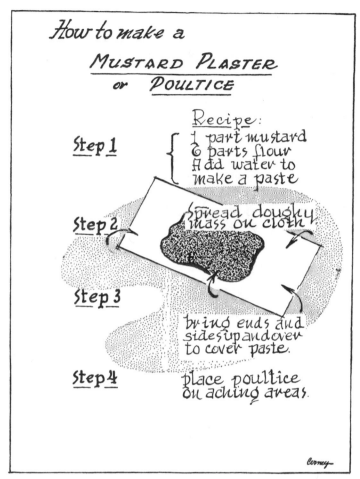

How to make a

MUSTARD PLASTER

or POULTICE

Step 1 {
Recipe:
1 part mustard
6 parts flour
Add water to
make a paste

Step 2
spread doughy
mass on cloth.

Step 3
bring ends and
sides up and over
to cover paste.

Step 4
place poultice
on aching areas.

Cerney

Figure 26

dries. Apply constantly until the fever drops and the cough stops.

4. MASSAGE muscles of neck, shoulder, chest, and back.

5. WARM DRY AIR to sooth a dry cough (hair dryer) DO NOT USE MEDICATED STEAM or get into a steam bath. Remember that volatile oils rising from a vaporizer are irritants. The chronic bronchitis victim has enough of irritants. He needs to be soothed!

6. WARM FULL BATH (see Figure 16) followed by a quick cold shower once or twice daily.

7. HOT "X" PACK over the neck and chest twice daily. Change every 10 minutes or as it cools. (Review Figure 18.)

8. HOT LEMONADE on the hour or as necessary to relieve the cough.

9. PREVENTION:
    A. Maintain a dust-free room. Keep it dry and well-aired.
    B. Avoid all tobacco and alcohol and extremes of temperature
    C. Wear clothing that *breathes* even while being warm.

10. DIETARY CONTROLS
    A. Fluids internally in abundance (fruit, vegetable and water only).

ACUTE BRONCHITIS

Bronchitis may be roughly divided into *acute* and *chronic* classifications. This is not to make the story more complex, but rather to clarify the matter to determine the best treatment for each. For example, *the person with acute bronchitis should breathe moist air. The person with chronic bronchitis should have it dry* . . . and warm. If it's acute bronchitis that you have here's the way to handle it:—

STEPS TO TAKE:

1. COLD "X" PACK on the neck and chest. (Review

Figure 18.) Change on the half hour or as it cools and dries. Apply constantly until the fever drops and the coughing stops.

2. MOIST AIR may be achieved with a tea kettle. Keep it boiling on a hot plate. This not only humidifies the air, but cuts down the dust content. It also helps loosen the exudate in the nose, throat and chest.

3. DIETARY CONTROLS
    A. Fluids internally in abundance (fruit, vegetable, water).
    B. Light diet (broths, soups).

4. PHYSIOLOGICAL CONTROLS
    A. Keep bowels open and kidneys active.
    B. During acute attacks, remain in bed even though there is no fever. Keep the windows open.
    C. Avoid all smoke, dust, fumes.
    D. Avoid all extremes of heat, cold, or moisture!

HOW TO HALT
HEART PROBLEMS
and Start Living Again

Rosemary de L. is one of my pet patients. I say this because after she tried everything else for her heart problem, she became a convert to water therapy and was "cured." Rosemary had been to many physicians. One said she had asthma because she wheezed like a sick workhorse and had harsh pains in her chest. She'd cough and up would come foul sputum which relieved her. Along with all the rest of the examination, I found a host of signs that would verify his diagnosis. I also found a number of tender "ouch spots" over her lower ribs. I used rotary pressure on these trigger zones and wrapped her in an "X" pack. After an hour her "asthma" was gone!

STEPS TO TAKE:

1. "X" PACK, cold (applied as shown in Figure 18) is applied AFTER the trigger points on the lower chest have been sought out and given rotary pressure.

2. ICE BAG to be placed on the spinal area between the second and tenth thoracic vertebra. Thirty minutes daily, three times a week.

3. HEART APPLICATION in the form of a *hot compress to be placed on the left side of the neck.* To accomplish this, fold a face towel into six thicknesses, Saturate with hot water. Wring. Apply. This is a vagal (heart) nerve stimulus. Apply for 30 minutes every second day.

4. MASSAGE the abdomen, and upper back muscles.

5. WALK AWAY FROM ALL EXCITEMENT! It's YOUR LIFE. Simply refuse to get involved!

6. KEEP KIDNEYS AND BOWELS OPEN

7. DON'TS to develop:
    A. Don't eat heavily at any time.
    B. Don't smoke or drink alcoholic beverages.
    C. Don't engage in too active exercise demanding sustained effort.

**Supplementary Procedures
for Heart Treatment**

Treatment of the heart problem with hydrotherapy is relatively simple and certainly inexpensive. Despite the complexity of the various heart conditions the treatments with water are very specific. For example, hot foot and hand baths are excellent for relieving the pain of *angina pectoris*. As a victim of this problem, I can vouch for the effectiveness of heat on the extremities.

To this add hot packs over the heart area for one minute and a cold pack alternately for five minutes. Also of help is the rotary pressure on pressure points or "ouch spots" found on the lower chest and left arm. Palpitation and *tachycardia* (fast beating of the heart) may be relieved promptly by using an ice compress on the nape of the neck. At the same time place the feet in a bucket of cold water. Treatment time is approximately five minutes per session. Do it twice daily.

PLEURISY . . . *What It Is*
How to Cope With It

Pleurisy is a nasty problem to have and if you catch it before effusion takes place in the lungs you've got it whipped. After the effusion (water in lungs) takes place, the treatment is different. Cold is applied first *before* effusion sets in. *After* effusion place, heat is applied.

STEPS TO TAKE:

Before Effusion Takes Place

1. *"X" PACK* (Review Figure 18) on the chest. This is a cross binder that is applied firmly and yet does not constrict breathing. Change quickly as it warms. This cold pack should take 20 minutes to an hour to warm.

After Effusion Takes Place

1. HOT POULTICES (Review Figure 26) or bran bags must

be applied constantly over an area larger then the point of pain. Heat the bran in a bag in boiling water. When the contents ooze through the cloth mesh, the bag is ready.

2. HOT FOMENTS may also be used. Change wet toweling every 15 minutes. Heat of the wet towel may be fortified with an infrared lamp if you have one, or, with a hot water bottle or hot brick. Where an infrared lamp is used, keep it at least 18° from target.

3. COLD MOIST PACK—and here's the secret to this procedure—should be given at least once daily in conjunction with the heat therapy.

> *Note: If the foments or poultices are objectionable, the half or sitz bath (Figure 12) may be tolerated. Keep water temperature between 80° and 85°F. Sit in the bath tub. Rub extremities and chest and back mildly. When the half bath is administered before bedtime, make the water temperature 95° to 98°F.*

EMERGENCY CARE FOR PNEUMONIA

Pneumonia is not a local disease. It's a general systemic problem with its focus in the lungs. When body resistance is down, when the lungs, liver, kidneys, skin, or heart are not functioning normally, a particular bacteria called *pneumococcus* sets up housekeeping in the lung tissues. The signs and symptoms of this disease are complicated, but the simple way to attack the pneumococcus, and what it is doing to you, is with water therapy. It's modern magic in an old-fashioned way. Here are three techniques you can use:—

Technique 1

STEPS TO TAKE:

1. SECTIONAL ABLUTIONS three times daily from head

to foot. Remember that *ablution* means local application of cold water with friction rub. Each body part is exposed separately from under the blanket. Each part is covered after being treated and the next part exposed. In having someone administer this treatment, or doing it on yourself, you will find that it is very invigorating and you will want to do it again and again.

2. COLD COMPRESSES on the thorax (chest) are to be alternated with the sectional ablution. This treatment is especially good if the heart is weak and the pulse soft. Change the cold compress every half hour or as it becomes warm.

3. SUNNY, WELL-VENTILATED ROOM is best for bed rest. Room temperature should be maintained at about 50°-60°F. Have a back rest made available in bed to make for more comfortable turning.

OTHER METHODS FOR TREATING PNEUMONIA WITH WATER THERAPY

Technique 2

STEPS TO TAKE:

1. "X" PACK around the thorax (see figure 18). Saturate sheeting with cold water (50°-60°F), ring out excess and apply. Change as it warms (every 20 minutes approximately).

2. RETENTION ENEMA (Review Figure 9) twice daily to maintain blood fluid level and stimulate the vasomotor nerves and hasten sweating from the skin. Enema water is cold (50°F). Add one tablespoonful of salt to one quart of water.

3. FLUID DIET may consist of fruit juices and broth, but NOT MILK. Alcoholic beverages are of no value in pneumonia! If the heart is involved, keep a cold compress over the heart area to stimulate it.

Technique 3

STEPS TO TAKE:

1. COLD HALF-SITZ BATH may be used twice daily for ten minutes at a time. This is accompanied by cold affusions and brisk rubbing on the neck and back. Have a friend pour cold water (50°F) from a bucket down the spine. Follow this with a brisk rubbing down each side of the spinal column.

   Note: If Technique One gives you good results, don't bother with Techniques Two and Three.

2. HOT SALINE (salt) GARGLES (one tablespoonful table salt to one quart of hot water).

3. FRUIT JUICES LIBERALLY all day long.

Here's What to Do
When Expectoration Stops:

1. HOT POULTICES (See Figure 26). Hot mustard poultice or plaster is recommended here. Place on the chest. Renew when it cools. Follow the removal of the plaster with a cold water rub and wrap up in a warm blanket. Get into bed.

"SHINGLES"

The technical handle for "shingles" is *herpes zoster*. As far as you and I are concerned let's call it "shingles" and be done with it. The "authorities" are apt to call this problem an "infection caused by a virus." They say it's like the virus that causes chicken pox, and little eruptions in the skin pop up. However, the same problem may follow carbon-monoxide poisoning or a dose of arsenic. Sometimes it appears in uremia (toxic urine products that get into the system) or in pneumonia. In a patient of mine—Theron G.—it came from garden spray, and if I hadn't enquired into his habits, I never would have determined the cause. I'd have been confused and called it "virus." Theron is a champion rose grower and hybridizer. He uses a lot of chemical sprays. One of them contains arsenic. After each spraying, he develops chills and fever. He gets "sick to his stomach," "feels lousy," and about the fourth day a crop of little blisters pop up in a line along his lower ribs. He said the first time he had it, "It was awfully painful, lots of little blisters and burning pain." After that, the "attacks" were just straight pain in the same area. Luckily in his case, the pain wasn't persistent as it is with some folks and our therapy stopped it completely. Along with discontinuing the arsenic sprays, here's the simplified technique he followed—

STEPS TO TAKE:

Ice Therapy for Shingles

1. ICE THERAPY is simple to apply. Simply apply an ice cube to the offended area. Do it lightly, gently. Follow the line of the ribs back to the spinal column (not just over the blister area). On either side of the spinal column, make rotary motions with the ice. Then put your thumb into an area there that is very tender on pressure. Press vigorously. If you can't reach it, place a golf ball in position and lie on it for a slow five count. Release. Repeat at least three times. If properly treated, a pleasant relief will follow.

water
treatment
for the
BACK

---

chapter
6

Subjects covered:

Lumbago
Sacro-iliac pain
Sciatica

WATER TECHNIQUES FOR
KNOCKING OUT LUMBAGO

He Made a Comeback
After Having Given Up

King M. had a marvelous name but an undistinguished career. He lived an undistinguished life and worked at an undistinguished job. He was "folks" like you and me. But, when that low back pain hit him there was nothing undistinguished about it. Sometimes the pain was mild, a dull ache, with maybe an itinerant dragging feeling every now and then. Then would come a sharp jabbing pain climaxed by non-stop agony. Anything could start it off. It got so fractious he was afraid to blow his nose or to sneeze. If he got out of a chair, if he turned suddenly, stepped down off a curbstone, if he lifted something heavy, if something hit him in the back, that was it! King couldn't even participate in his nocturnal duties and his wife divorced him. Then, because he couldn't lift boxes in the plant shipping department—which was his job—he was fired. When I saw him, his back was rigid, muscles pulled up hard and tight. To see if he might be fibbing I asked him to pick up an x-ray film which I had "accidently" dropped on the floor. He couldn't. All he could do was bend at the knees. Low back involvements—like King's—may be due to faulty posture, weak muscles, infections, exposure to wetness and cold, or even a too strenuous occupation. The back muscles and their surrounding soft tissues become inflamed. They contracted. Presto . . . *lumbago*! If you have had this low back discomfort you know what King went through. If you want to know what brought him out of his disaster area here's the process that brought him quick, long lasting relief. In addition to the *Relaxation Bath, Ice Packs, Muscle Massage,* study the how-to-do-its on the *"Wet Sheet Pack"* and the French Dr. Gustave

Monod's *"Friction Rub."* They will play an important role in your health from this book on.

STEPS TO TAKE:

> *First*
> *Night*

    1. RELAXATION BATH (Review Figure 26 followed by—

    2. ICE PACKS or "SCOTCH DOUCHE" (cold bathtub spray) or, an "ice-cube rub" over the "trigger points" (ouch spots) that you find—or a friend finds—on your back. To be remembered is that *no matter what the cause of the back pain, you can relieve that pain with cold therapy*! Apply the ice pack, or the ice-cube rub, immediately over the point of pain. Inscribe small circles if you are using an ice cube. At no time keep the ice on so long that the skin blanches. If you can not get at your own back, have a friend use the ice-cube technique on you, or, fill a sandwich bag with crushed ice and lie back on it.

                Here's an Important
                Point to Remember:

    The big secret to learn in inflammation of muscles (as in lumbago) is that—(a) If muscles are treated with cold procedures in the early stage of injury good results are almost immediate. This is called the "acute stage". However, the secret to home therapy for chronically contracted and hurting muscles lies in (b) heat plus cold water friction.[1]

    3. MUSCLES MASSAGE (after ice therapy) should al-

---

[1]Heat may be derived from a full relaxation bath, a half-sitz bath, from a tea kettle (steam) or over a hot air register in your home. Hot foments should be re-applied every 10 to 20 minutes. Follow immediately with cold friction rubs. (See the amazing Monod "Friction Rub.")

ways include muscles of the thighs and buttocks as well as the muscles of the low back. Do it gently but firmly. In addition to the massage, stroke the back with a sponge full of hot water. Beneath your very fingertips, these angrily contracted muscles will begin to relax.

> *Second*
> *Night*

4. WET SHEET PACK (¾ or full pack) to be used cold on alternate nights in place of the ice pack, ice-cube rub or the cold Scotch douche. Become adept at this "wet pack" technique because it will be worth a million dollars in health and saved doctor bills for you and your family. To give you a better understanding of applying a wet sheet here's how to handle—

THE THREE-QUARTER PACK

> *NOTE: One exception distinguishes the ¾ pack from the Full Pack: –it does not enclose the arms. The arms remain free under the bedclothes. This is recommended for those people who have a fear of being closed in (claustrophobia). The ¾ pack is applied from the armpits down and is indicated for all back problems as well as for arthritis, rheumatism, fever, insomnia, neurasthenia and all toxic problems (fever etc.).*

Significant Facts about ¾ and Full Packs and Their Wonderful Values

Powerful elimination factors are at work in this process of natural healing. The body eliminates waste. As the skin becomes activated by the intimate impact of cold, the blood supply immediately in and under the skin is chased away. This is followed by a complete new blood supply rushing in to take its place. It's

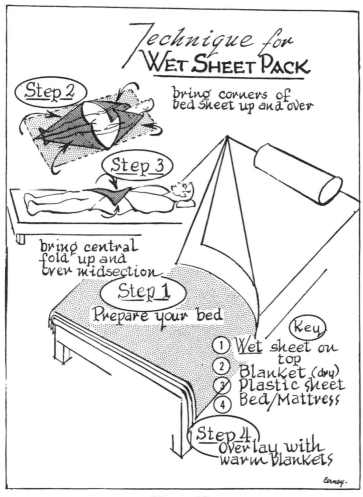

Figure 27

action and reaction, and the pack begins to warm as the body radiates its own heat. This sends the internal body fever—if fever is present—externally. What you provide in the wet sheet pack, then, is an escape. You have helped the pores of the skin to relax. You have permitted perspiration to break loose and when this occurs the "fever is broken."

Wet packs quite often are applied locally over a single joint, or around the throat for tonsillitis, etc., but the full and ¾ packs are more therapeutically effective. When local problems show a great deal of poisonous waste (infection), as in a "cold in the head," the ¾ pack is best. There is no ailment for which a "pack" cannot be used. Plainly and simply, it decongests acute and chronic problems and aids toxic elimination and that's the significant fact.

Special Notes
on Pack Application:

1. Apply all packs in a warm room.

2. Remove the pack when the warming reaction DOES NOT take place!

3. *If you are fasting* DO NOT use the wet pack in any form!

4. Shower thoroughly after a good sweating session. Your body will be covered with body waste.

5. Wash and air the sheeting immediately! It, too, is foul with body waste.

Supplementary Reminders
in Lumbago Care

(1) Remove the cause! (2) Improve your posture! (3) Exercise to strengthen the muscles of the back (4) Apply local poultices where local heat is desirable. (5) Where local cold compresses are applied, renew them every 10 to 20 minutes or as they warm. Follow three or four local wet sheet packs with rubbing and kneading of muscles. In chronic myositis (inflamed muscles), utilize hot packs followed by a quick cold shower or cold water rub and a brisk toweling.

SACRO-ILIAC PAIN
AND HOW TO HANDLE IT

Sacro-iliac pain is usually found on one side of the low

back. Its pain may extend down the sciatic nerve into the extremity. It is usually caused by a separation of the joint between the sacrum bone and one of the pelvic bones called the ilium. Ligaments that bind that joint may be stretched, sprained or strained. The joint may get out of its normal alignment. There are many causes for this condition. Too much lying in bed may bring it on. "Easy" chairs may start it off. Broken arches or a short leg distorting the pelvis may precipitate the problem. Faulty posture is a contributing agent. Getting up out of bed, or even sneezing, may start the pain. Bending at the waist or leaning sidewise may do it and the person with the problem quickly learns what to do and what not to do to prevent it from happening. Cal H. had such a problem.

Storekeeper Finds Way to Combat Low Back Pain

Cal H. was just taking an item off the shelf in his grocery store when pain shot through his low back and thigh. It was a disabling pain. Two of his clerks had to help him to my office. After examination and treatment he was given the following regimen to follow: He did. No reoccurrences.

STEPS TO TAKE:

1. COLD COMPRESSES are placed over the sacro-iliac joints (See Figure 28) for the first two days. Thereafter, use alternate hot and cold packs if the pain persists.

2. MASSAGE all muscles of the low back and thighs. DO NOT MASSAGE OVER THE SICK JOINT!

3. BED REST is of no advantage without resting the involved sciatic nerve. To accomplish this in bed, place a strip of plywood (4' x 6') under the matress to reduce the amount of "give." Place a pillow under your knees for added comfort when lying on your back.

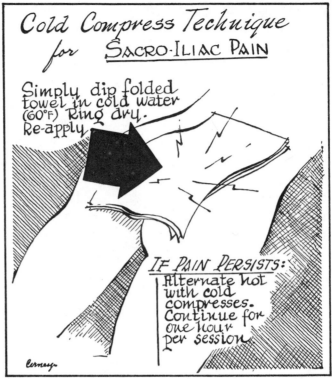

Figure 28

4. MUSTARD PLASTER (Review Figure 26) over the involved sacro-iliac joint.

5. NO-NO's: —avoid all positions or conditions that aggravate the problem.

SCIATICA!
*Special Water Controls and
How to Handle It*

**Race Driver Gets Back to
Driving After On-the-Spot
Water Treatment**

Like the word arthritis, the word *sciatica* is merely a symptom. It is not a disease. It indicates only that the sciatic nerve trunk has become inflamed or that there is some interference with the passage of nerve impulses somewhere along its course, or, at such points as it exits from the spinal cord. Pressure on this nerve is probably one of its worst offenders, although reflexes, diseases of local joints, chilling, direct blows, tumors, spinal punctures for anesthesia, etc. may all cause, or contribute to, this particular pain. In other words there are many causes.

John R's leg "went dead" when his prostate enlarged and his sciatic nerve sustained compression on it. Layne P.'s leg-pain began with sitting constantly perched on the edge of an architect's stool. Then there was a race driver Danny L. Danny developed "automobile sciatica" from spending all his time in the bucket seat of his speedster. Truck drivers get the same thing. Pregnancies may start the same kind of pain. The point is that *pressure triggers the problem.*

When Danny L. showed up at the office, he complained of stabbing or burning pain. He said that sometimes it felt like a knife ripping through his thigh and back. Sometimes the pain went down his leg to his heel. In your own case, if you've ever had sciatica, you know what Danny went through. Even more than this *you can put your finger on the exact spot where it hurts and this is the secret to treating yourself at home!* X marks the spot! This is the hypersensitive area that you treat with water therapy.

One warning note before treatment begins: —*Find the cause!* Remember that no matter what treatment is rendered if you don't get rid of the cause—the original irritant to that sciatic nerve—the problem will start up once more.

STEPS TO TAKE:

Acute Stage

1. COLD COMPRESSES along the course of the inflamed

nerve are applied even while keeping the balance of the body warm with blankets. (Do NOT use any massage procedures in the acute or beginning stages!)

2. IMMOBILIZE THE AFFECTED LIMB with pillows on each side of the limb and one under the knee.

3. DIETARY CONTROLS: eat rich food unless you have rheumatism or gout along with your sciatica. This is one of the few times I advocate "rich" foods for anything. In addition, add Vitamin B complex to your diet.

4. INTESTINAL LAVAGE (Review Figure 9). Use cold water only in a continuous flow. Lie on the side of the accentuated pain. Do this daily. The water may be mildly soapy (do *not* use a detergent soap—use Ivory)

| *Chronic* |
| *Stage* |

1. HOT FULL BATH: After the first ten minutes submerged start your legs moving. Keep them moving under water. Maintain 105°F temperature for 30 minutes. Follow with a quick cold shower, a brisk rubdown and into bed. Relax. Sleep for two or more hours.

2. MASSAGE may be used at this point if done mildly. *Massage* is to be *applied TWO HOURS AFTER a hot full bath* and relaxation in a warm bed. Massage all muscles of the back, abdomen and both lower extremities. *DO NOT massage OVER ANY AREA OF PAIN!* Begin nerve stretching routine by gently bending the leg and then extending it, straightening it, and in straightened position extend it just that little bit extra.

> NOTE: *Remember that in ALL cases—acute or chronic— FIND THE CAUSE! Then prevent it from reoccurring! An ounce of prevention is still worth a pound of cure in sciatica as in every other health problem . . . even in an age of miracle drugs!*

water

treatment

for the

ABDOMEN

(Alimentary and Urinary Systems)

---

chapter

7

Subjects covered:

ANUS	Hemorrhoids		Excess Gastric acidity
APPENDIX	Appendicitis		Flatulence
			Gastralgia
BLADDER	Anuria		Gastric Juice (lack of)
	Bedwetting		Indigestion
	Cystitis		Nausea
	Nephritis		Ulcer (duodenal)
DIGESTIVE	Colitis	LIVER	Biliousness
ORGANS	Constipation		Cholecystitis
	Diarrhea		Gall stones
	Dilated Stomach		Yellow Jaundice

WHAT DO DO ABOUT
ANAL HEMORRHOIDS

One of the most efficient methods for relief of hemorrhoids is the *"T" Strap*. Where hemorrhoids are of somewhat new origin this excellent treatment causes them to contract and disappear. The cold wet pack also acts as a styptic and stops bleeding. A cold compress may also be placed over the sacrum and coccyx (tailbone) to strengthen the shutting-off of bleeders in the rectal area.

Hemorrhoids are at no time totally local. They may be the result of toxic waste in the circulation, back pressure from the liver on the portal circulation, constipation and high blood pressure. They may be an occupational hazard from constant sitting (truckdrivers), or from straining at stool. But no matter what the cause, the cold "T" Strap (see Figure 29) is the treatment of choice.

A relative of mine we'll call Anna M. had rectal hemorrhoids. They hung out like a bunch of grapes. They itched. They burned. They drove her frantic. Since she was so obese I advised her that the best thing for her was surgery. Anna wouldn't buy this idea at all. To appease her demand for help I taught her how to apply the "T" Strap, what to do about her diet, how to get her bowels to move gently, and how to place an ice bag over her tailbone. Two weeks later, Anna came into the office glowing. That big woman hugged and kissed me in the crowded waiting room until I was embarrassed to death. She beamed as she told the world about her problem and how it was conquered. I didn't feel that I had much to do with it—just a little guidance—but in that cold water "T" Strap, and digestive controls was the hand of God. Nature still remains the best doctor after all.

STEPS TO TAKE:

1. "T" STRAP (Figure 29)

2. PERINEAL DOUCHE (Figure 30)

3. COLD HIP SITZ BATH (Review Figure 12)

Do the above three procedures on alternate days. Concurrently apply—

4. COLD COMPRESSES (Review Figure 1) on sacrum

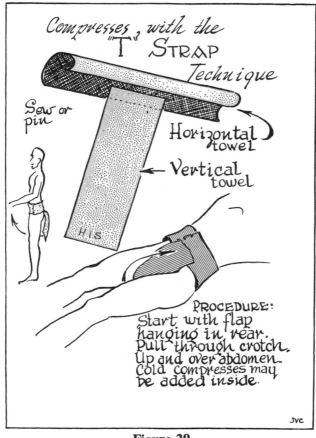

Compresses, with the "T" Strap Technique

Sew or pin

Horizontal towel

Vertical towel

H.is

PROCEDURE:
Start with flap hanging in rear. Pull through crotch. Up and over abdomen. Cold compresses may be added inside.

JVC

Figure 29

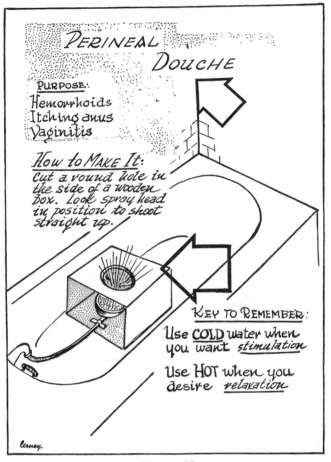

Figure 30

and rectal area. Re-cool it as it warms. Apply it for an hour before bedtime.

5. MASSAGE deeply into all soft tissues around the tailbone and low back area. Be gentle.

6. NO EXERCISE. Avoid all forms of manual activity until healing takes place. No heavy lifting, no long walks, no horse or bicycle riding, or even long rides in planes, trains, trucks, trains, planes, or buses.

7. DIETARY CONTROLS:
   A. DON'T eat highly seasoned foods

    B. DON'T drink alcoholic beverages, coffee, tea or cola drinks

    C. DON'T eat foods contributing to constipation and/or hard bowel movements.

    D. DO eat easily digested foods (broths, soups).

    E. DO drink copiously of water or juices.

8. HYGIENIC CONTROLS:

    A. *Wash anus* after each voiding. Use soap and water or baby oil. *Note:* Do not use colored tissues. (*Dye in the paper too often starts an inflammatory condition* and local poisoning)

    B. *Evacuate bowels daily.* Go the moment you get the impulse. Make it your personal rule to let nothing interfere. When you have to go, GO!

HOW TO RELIEVE
APPENDICITIS
UNTIL THE DOCTOR COMES

I was stepping out of a north woods fishing lodge, with all gear on, ready for a great day, when the lodge manager stopped me at the door. He was excited. There was a man in 302, he said, with pain in his belly. I looked longingly out at the lake, turned and went back to 302. Glad I did. John Smith (we'll call him that because he's a high-line government official) was in agony. His face was haggard. His abdomen was as hard as a rock. I managed to learn that the night before he didn't feel much like eating. He had been nauseated and had some discomfort around his navel. He vomited a little and during the night the pain localized in his lower right side.

It became a very sharp pain. When he sneezed or coughed, it nearly cut him in half.

I had my suspicions about the problem but followed my examination through. My suspicions were wrong! It was not appendicitis! The symptoms were the same but after checking up through the rectum I found a tumorous mass in the lower right abdomen. I felt there was no possibility of the appendix rupturing or peritonitis setting in so water therapy was begun immediately until we could get a seaplane and fly him out.[1]

The whole point is that what *appeared* to look like appendicitis was NOT! On the other hand, no matter what the cause of that lower right abdominal pain, the treatment is the same . . . cold water therapy! The following reveals the procedure used effectively on Mr. Smith. It can do just as well for you.

STEPS TO TAKE:

1. COLD WET COMPRESSES (Review Figure 1) to be continued over a 12-hour period. Cover entire abdomen. In this particular case DO NOT USE ICE! Saturate your toweling, wring excess cold water out, apply, remove and re-apply as it warms, on the back, place—

2. COLD PACK OR ICE BAG over the mid and low back.

Note: Here's your key to proper use of abdominal packs: —THE MOMENT PAIN SUBSIDES IN THE BACK AND BELLY you can replace the cold packs with HOT PACKS ON THE SOLAR PLEXUS and appendix areas! Hot packs are applied in the same manner as cold packs or compresses over the belly.

3. DO NOT TAKE LAXATIVES, cathartics or purgatives under any circumstance during this type of hurt in the abdomen.

4. WARM SOAPSUDS ENEMA may be used to relieve the lower bowel. (90°-95°F) However, *where the tummy muscles have become rigid DO NOT USE AN ENEMA!*

5. THIRST may be quenched with cold water.

6. ABSOLUTE BED REST

---

[1]In appendicitis, or other similar types of abdominal pain, the purpose of hydrotherapy is to (1) quell inflammation, (2) relieve tension of muscles, and, (3) assist absorption of poisonous exudates. COLD is always the procedure of demand, not choice. This is always my choice before thinking of surgery.

7. FULL RELAXATION BATH (Review Figure 16) (cold) after the initial pain begins to subside. In John Smith's case, because there were no bathtubs in the lodge, I took him down to the lake and sat him ribs deep in water. He thought I was crazy but he did it. Everybody else thought I was crazy. The proof, however, was in the pudding. We never did have to call for that seaplane to get him back to civilization. Months later I received a communication from him in Washington. He was feeling fit as a fiddle. Specialists had confirmed my diagnosis. The tumor proved to be benign.

8. MASSAGE THE MUSCLES of the low back, upper back and neck. DO NOT MASSAGE THE ABDOMEN at any time!

9. When in doubt see your doctor immediately.

KIDNEY and URINARY PROBLEMS

Anuria

Bedwetting

Cystitis

Nephritis

CONQUERING ANURIA
with Nature's Most Magic Remedy

Anuria is not something with which to play and make jokes

about. It is nothing to scoff at or hide. Outside the fact that the bladder is not voiding there may be very little else to indicate the problem that's going on in the urinary system.

In addition to not being able to urinate, Tim H. complained of headache. He said that he had a pain in his low back and that now and again he felt like vomiting. Other than that . . . nothing! In Tim's case, I found that an enlarged prostate was obstructing the passage of urine. In Mrs. W's case, it came after she'd had a bad bout of fever picked up in South America. In Francie M.'s case, her anuria started after she'd had a bad automobile accident and was thrown from her car. She went into shock. In all cases urine was suppressed. Then there was Dolph T.'s case.

A Plasterer Cures Inability to Urinate with Hydrotherapy

Dolph T. had been in the construction business for years. He's an A-1 plasterer. Like a lot of other plasterers he has a bladder problem. There are many reasons for bladder problems. Nerves may be involved. Tumors may cause it. A blow may start it off. Alcoholic beverages may be a contributing factor. In Dolph's case it was a blow. He fell off scaffolding in an apartment project. Because of spinal fracturing he had to go into a cast. He urinated less and less until only the overflowing from his overcrowded bladder was being voided . . . at the wrong times. His odor was awful and he couldn't help it. When he finally got back on the job, he kept changing uniforms but the dribbling continued to stain him. His bladder was simply toneless. Under normal circumstance, after such an injury, the individual, within six weeks after an accident—and as nerves repair—is automatically restored back to normal. In Dolph's case it wasn't. He had cystoscopic studies, catheterizations, x-rays, drugs, the whole bit, and he was getting a little desperate. That's when I saw him for the first time professionally. After studying his total picture, I started him on the following regimen that brought him king-size relief. No more embarrassments. He's back to normal once more.

> *NOTE: Because no kind of treatment is of value until in-flammation and swelling are gone from the kidneys, all proce-dures must be designed to accomplish just this. For this reason the following are recommended:–*

STEPS TO TAKE:

1. HOT COLONIC IRRIGATION (enema) (Review Figure 9). Retain water as hot as tolerable. Solution = one tablespoon-ful of table salt to one quart of water. Re-apply every two hours.

2. LEMONADE—3 ounces every 30 minutes for a week.

3. HOT FOMENTATIONS (See Figure 31)—Anoint the body part to be treated with olive oil before applying a hot

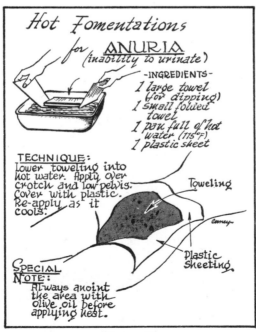

Figure 31

fomentation. The foment package is simply made. Use two towels: one small, one large. Fold the smaller towel in fourths. Center it on the larger towel. While holding the ends of the large towel lower the central area into a bucket of hot water (115°F). Squeeze dry. Apply hot wet section over the low pelvis. Lap the free or dry ends of the large towel up and over the small towel. Cover this with a piece of plastic and lie down in bed. Cover yourself well and let the fomentation do its work.

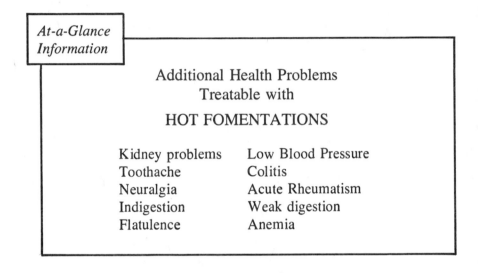

At-a-Glance Information

Additional Health Problems
Treatable with

HOT FOMENTATIONS

Kidney problems	Low Blood Pressure
Toothache	Colitis
Neuralgia	Acute Rheumatism
Indigestion	Weak digestion
Flatulence	Anemia

BED WETTING
AND HOW TO STOP IT

Little Tommy F. was born with weak sphincter muscles in his bladder. He couldn't control them. Some folks acquire this problem. Usually bed wetting starts around the ages of five or six and its causes may be many. The rectum may be involved. Cause may be in the vagina, the kidneys, malnutrition or anemia. A feeling of insecurity may trigger it. Worms may do it to children. Broken down feet have been known to be a cause. Because of this, *the first necessity is to remove the cause!* The irritability that triggers it has to be eliminated. In all cases, however, water therapy, in my experience, proves to be the effective agent in coping with the problem with children as well as with adults. Here's the procedure I used on Tommy to strengthen his weak bladder-control sphincters. The same treatment is good for bed wetting from almost any cause.

STEPS TO TAKE:

1. COLD WET COMPRESSES (Review Figure 1). Apply layers of cold wet toweling on the mid and low back for 30 minutes before bedtime. Twice weekly. To this add:—

2. COLD FOOT BATH or WATER TREADING (review Figure 5) Treat water or soak in cold water bath (60°F) for one minute *only*. Follow with a brisk toweling and get into bed.

3. ELEVATE THE FOOT OF THE BED (for nighttime sleeping).

4. DIETARY CONTROLS: Largest meal to be eaten at noontime. Only a light lunch in the evening. Avoid all salt, sweets, and liquids after 4:00 PM.

5. PRESSURE POINT CONTROL:
   A. *Thumb pressure* in the lumbar area. You can locate tenderness zones in the low back immediately by probing along the spinal column. Once located, sink a knuckle in and hold it.

6. THE AWARD SYSTEM when used on children should take the place of threats, spankings, or reprimands. With "nervous" children don't permit them to get fatigued before retiring. Teach them to evacuate before bedtime. Reward them for good results but NEVER CHASTISE THEM! It only compounds the problem!

7. REMOVE THE CAUSE: —excitement, tension, illness, excesses in anything and everything.

8. HOT SITZ BATHS (Review Figure 12) may follow the application of the cold compress procedure after the first week of

water therapy. Temperature—105°F, for ten minutes, followed by two minutes of cold showering. Dry briskly and go to bed. Repeat nightly and each morning for four weeks. Results will be very much noticeable.

9. "T" STRAP (Review Figure 29). A cold "T" Strap may be used in place of the cold compress or foment on the abdomen and pelvis.

HOW TO BEAT THOSE ANNOYING BLADDER PROBLEMS

If you have ever been victimized by cystitis, you know it's no fun. Cystitis is an inflammation of the urinary bladder. Bacteria, medication, food, or a direct blow to the abdomen may cause it to happen. It happened that way with karate student Jeanne T. As a result, she dribbled night and day. In addition to dribbling she started to have pain during urination. Sometimes the pain was deep in her pelvis. Sometimes it radiated up into her abdomen. Sometimes down her thighs. She had had no relief from various kinds of treatment until she started water therapy. After the following program went into effect, she reported that her backache had disappeared, that she was no longer going sleepless at night, that she didn't have a constant urge to urinate, that the discomfort in her legs had stopped. Most of all she was happy the "cold feeling in her spine" was gone. For the same kind of results here are the—

STEPS TO TAKE:

1. COLD WET COMPRESSES (Review Figure 1) for the first two weeks over the lumbar and sacral area (low back and tailbone). Where this does not bring relief follow with a cold *"T" Strap* (See Figure 29) or *Scotch Douche* shower bath (Review Figure 15).

2. ICE WATER ENEMA followed by—

3. HOT HIP SITZ BATH (105° to 115°F) for 20 minutes, once weekly, three times per day, or, hot foments over the lower abdomen and pubes.

4. REST IN BED with hips and legs elevated.

5. MASSAGE ABDOMEN deeply but gently.

6. DIETARY CONTROLS
   A. *Bland diet* (no heavy foods of any kind!) soups. (No starch or protein solids)
   B. *Drink water copiously.* Peppermint tea is also excellent.

7. COLONIC IRRIGATIONS to keep the bowels open. (Review Figure 9).

POSITIVE HOME REMEDIES
FOR NEPHRITIS
(Inflamed Kidneys)

When your kidneys are inactive something else has to take over their duty of excretion. The secret to "bad kidney function" lies in water therapy used to open the ducts of the skin in getting rid of kidney and other body waste.

A Bus Driver Finds
Relief from Nephritis

Bus Driver Joey D. had nephritis and he had no idea that it was affecting his blood pressure or causing his feet to swell. His case of acute nephritis hit suddenly. It came a week after he had had a bad infection in his mouth. He had a bad headache, 101°F fever, vomiting, nausea and very little urine was voided. The very thought of food made him feel worse. Because his kidneys weren't working—and because his skin was not letting body waste out—the water backed up in his system. His feet began to swell. His eyelids puffed, and because his heart had a greater job to do to circumvent the problem, his blood pressure went up 40 points over his usual normal 120/80. The little urine he made was smoky and dark. Another thing he complained of was pain in his flanks. If you have any of this the following program is just for you:—

ACUTE NEPHRITIS

STEPS TO TAKE:

1. HALF HOT SITZ BATH (Review Figure 12) temperature—102°-105°F for 30 minutes. Maintain a cold compress on top of your head while sitting in the tub. Drink as much lemonade as possible during the treatment. Repeat this bath four times daily for one week. If the half bath does not get results, use the *hot blanket* (also known as *"Tent Sitz"*) (See Figure 36). Sweating will start immediately.

> **SPECIAL NOTE: If you have a heart problem**
> **DO NOT USE THIS METHOD!**

2. FRICTION RUB (Check index for "Salt Glow" and "Monod friction rub").

3. DRINK WATER and fruit juices copiously. At least three ounces every half hour.

4. AVOID ALL DRAFTS, air-conditioned places and cold wet weather.

5. KEEP YOUR BEDROOM WARM (avoid all possibilities of chilling).

6. NO SOLID FOODS until the acute stage of nephritis is over. Remain primarily on milk and fruit and vegetable juices, soup and broth.

CHRONIC NEPHRITIS

Winnie W. came in complaining of headache, weakness, digestive disturbances, dry skin, and the fact that she was having trouble with her vision. She complained about her fingers getting white and tingly, and that at times she was dizzy, nauseated and constantly tired. Sometimes she was even stuporous and the problem got so bad she had to quit her job. Her biggest complaint was that her problem was interfering with her sex life.

Winnie already had seven children. She also had a husband who was an alcoholic. Two of her teenage daughters, unmarried, were pregnant. Her oldest son was in the detention home for lifting hub caps. Her blood pressure went up, up, up. She was constantly urinating and when she got another job on the night shift of an office building clean-up crew she spent most of her time running to the john. Because of constantly running to the toilet, she was accused of "goofing off" from her job and dismissed. When I saw her, her eyelids were nearly swollen shut with edema. She was anemic, pale. Her morale was at an all time low. I laid out a program for her to follow. She did. She recovered and you can do the same. Here's how:—

STEPS TO TAKE:

1. HOT COMPRESSES (Review Figure 1) over the entire low back for 30 minutes per session. Repeat twice daily. First, anoint the skin with oil before applying the hot pack. After improvement starts, and you are feeling better, start using these hot packs three times weekly. Instead of 30 minutes per treatment, extend the treatment time to one hour.

2. HOT FULL OR RELAXING BATH (Review Figure 16) twice weekly. Remain in the hot tub only until such time as the sweat breaks out on your forehead. Take a quick cold shower. Rub down with a rough towel and go to bed.

3. MASSAGE all back muscles and down over the sacrum (tailbone). Massage deeply, but gently, into the abdomen.

4. EXERCISE regularly outdoors. Dry climates are best. Wear clothing to maintain body warmth.

5. DIETARY CONTROLS. Light diet (soup, broth) with a lot of other liquids (vegetable and fruit juices and water).NO MEAT! To this diet add stewed prunes, baked apples, rice pudding and plenty of milk if you can tolerate it. AVOID: all seasoned foods, pastries, alcohol, tea, coffee, "soft" drinks, spices and drugs. DO USE (as progress begins to show) corn bread, tapioca, rice, macaroni, fresh vegetables, butter, bacon, potatoes, olive oil, white meat of chicken, fresh fish, clams, fresh beef (small portion) young mutton, buttermilk, ginger ale, lemonade, oranges, and apples.

(Alimentary System)
STOMACH
and BOWELS

Colitis

Constipation

Diarrhea

Dilated stomach

Excess gastric acidity

Flatulence

Gastralgia

Gastric juices (lack of)

Indigestion
Nausea
Ulcer (duodenal, gastric)

HOW TO OVERCOME
COLITIS
(Inflamed Bowel)

Bacteria, allergies, and even emotions contribute to colitis. One of the worst offenders is the very life we lead. We pay the price for abnormal tensions if we don't know how to handle them. *Colitis* means an "irritable colon." The problem is compounded intermittently by constipation and diarrhea. It may go on to ulceration and usually happens to folks in their 20's, 30's and 40's.

James M. had this problem. He said he didn't even know when it began. Suddenly, there it was: —constipation alternating with diarrhea, loss of appetite, slight fever at night. He had headaches, insomnia, abdominal discomfort, loss of weight. Sometimes he felt nauseous and wanted to vomit. Sometimes there was mucous in his feces. Sometimes even blood. But outside there was nothing physically (externally) other than some hemorrhoids and itching at the anus.

In my experience with colitis patients I find they are usually the "nervous" type. Sometimes people with a weak constitution tend to get colitis. Sometimes it may be caused by an inadequate diet or harsh laxatives. Irritating drugs may bring it on. Diets heavy in starch and light in vegetables and alkaline fruits may trigger it. Worst offenders are nerve-depressing foods and drugs. In James M's case, we started him on the following program, and within weeks—for a problem that he'd had for many years—he had almost instant relief. I'm not saying you will get the same sensational results but if you stick to the following health rules you will achieve the same great feeling of well-being as did he.

STEPS TO TAKE:

1. Alternate HOT-COLD HIP SITZ BATHS daily. (Review Figure 12).

2. FASTING on water and diluted fruit juices—up to a gallon of liquid a day—for three to six days.

3. INTESTINAL LAVAGE (daily) with tepid water (85°F) to keep the bowels cleaned out. DO NOT USE LAXATIVES WHEN CONSTIPATED!

4. ALL-MILK DIET to follow your three day water fast. You may drink as much as two gallons of milk a day. Repeat this diet daily for seven days. Be sure that the milk is lukewarm. Sip it. Don't gulp!

5. HOT FOMENTATIONS (Review Figure 31) on the abdomen before bedtime if pain is present. Always anoint the skin of the abdomen with olive oil before placing the hot foment down on the skin. *When there is no pain or discomfort in the abdomen USE COLD PACKS* on the belly nightly. One hour.

6. HOT FULL RELAXATION BATH (Review Figure 16) may begin after the first week of the above treatments. The full tub should be taken twice weekly. Add Epsom salts (two handsful) per tub. Remain in the tub 30 to 60 minutes, or, until sweat breaks out of the forehead (115°F). Follow with a quick cold shower and a fast friction rub with the hands or coarse toweling. This therapy releases body waste. It helps especially in reducing body acidity. Take your relaxation bath before bedtime. This is excellent for those folks knotted up with tensions from the day's activities.

7. DIETARY CONTROLS should follow immediately when the milk-diet stops. Here's the diet to follow: —

FOOD CONTROL
FOR COLITIS

Breakfast: fruit juices and oatmeal (milk and honey)

Mid-morning: fruit juices

Lunch: lettuce salad with grated raw carrots, chopped
raw spinach, onions, cabbage (use lemon
dressing or olive oil)

Mid-afternoon: fruit juice or weak tea

Dinner: salad (as at noon) yoghurt, fresh fruit.

DIETING PERIOD for Colitis: 10-20 days

CONTRAINDICATIONS:
DON'T EAT excess starches,
DON'T EAT Meats, fried foods, white sugar, spices.
Avoid everything with white flour.

Note: Where mucous colitis is chronic it is advisable
to repeat your milk fasting procedure at
monthly intervals . . . or less . . . as desired.

HOW TO RESTORE REGULARITY
AND STOP CONSTIPATION

John M.K. had as many physical complaints as Sears and
Roebuck has catalogs. As I took his history and the story of his
current problems, the report swelled to volume size. I listened in
amazement. I didn't want to believe that this man could ache
from head to toe in such a manner, that maybe he was stretching
it a little or had been reading some medical books too diligently.
Then I remembered a professor at college saying that *most
human diseases begin in the gut.* He went on to explain how

headaches, coated tongue, irritability, joint aches, muscle aches, abdominal discomfort, "heartburn and gas" were just a few of the problems that take place when the organs of the abdomen are not doing their job. Because the duty of the large bowel is to absorb fluid, it also absorbs waste from that bowel and as long as that bowel is not cleansed of its contents this waste is absorbed directly into the blood stream and from there all over the body. Physical parts automatically rebel against the presence of this poison in the form of arthritis (joints), myositis (muscles) and muscle cramps, poor eyesight, headaches, etc. . . . and adding drugs or other chemicals to this septic tank only adds to the problem. I never forgot that lecture and as I listened to John M.K. I suspected that he was right! Maybe his chronic constipation WAS the cause of it all!

It's true that constipation has other causes. The cause may be emotional. It may be the result of long sitting during travel, from dietary indiscretion and inadequate digestive apparatus, drinking insufficient amounts of liquid, lack of exercise, overuse of laxatives and/or purges. As a national American disease, constipation, and its sometimes-alternate diarrhea, results in inflammation of the bowel called *colitis*. This inflammation may be due to too many starches in the diet, too much sugar, too much tension and too many failures to respond to the "call" to evacuate the bowels. Too often, chronic constipation resists accepted medical treatment and surgery is used. In my estimation this is a desperate and unnecessary move in most cases as we have proven consistently over the years. John M.K. was such a case.

After a thorough examination looking for bowel strictures, adhesions, fissures, fistulae, diverticulae or pouches, hemorrhoids and other factors that may contribute to the inability to evacuate, I checked to see if John had a spastic or atonic colon and this is *your* key! If your physician tells you you have a *spastic colon* (where the bowel wall is all contracted and knotted up), you use following Technique 1. If he informs you that you have an *atonic colon* (without mobility or tone) (stretched out like an old innertube), then you use Technique 2. Here's how it's done: —

Technique 1

HOW TO HANDLE
SPASTIC BOWEL CONDITIONS

STEPS TO TAKE:

1. INTESTINAL LAVAGE (105°-110°F), one quart of hot water in a family size douche bag permitted to enter. Hold. Rest. Repeat with a second quart if you can take it. Evacuate. Go to bed. Rest. Olive oil may be added to the water (½ cupful per quart of water. You may also add one tablespoonful of table salt.)

Technique 2:

HOW TO HANDLE
ATONIC BOWEL CONDITIONS

STEPS TO TAKE:

1. WARM FULL BATHS (85°F) (Review Figure 16) once daily for 10 minutes per session. Followed by—

2. COLD ABLUTIONS are applied with a brisk hand rubbing of the entire body with cold water while standing in the bathtub—or you may use a sharp shower (cold).

3. COLD ABDOMINAL PACK before bedtime—or—

4. INTESTINAL LAVAGE (colonic irrigation) cold, applied every second evening with water temperature starting at 85°F and decreasing gradually to 60°F. An alternate to this is the—

5. COLD HALF SITZ BATH (Review Figure 12) with brisk rubbing of the abdomen.

6. DRINKING WATER or fruit juices, copiously, is required all day long. At no time should water therapy be deemed the total answer to the problem of chronic constipation. It is NOT! It should be combined properly with proper hygiene, proper diet, and total better living which may be often just the total opposite of the life you have been leading . . . the very kind of life that brought the problem on in the first place.

7. FRICTION RUB (See Monod *"Friction Rub"* or *"Salt Glow"* in the Index.

**Supplementary
Technique 3:**

EUROPEAN TECHNIQUE
FOR CHRONIC CONSTIPATION

1. *Cold Hip Sitz Bath each morning*

2. *Alternate hot/cold sitz bath* (each night)

3. *Epsom salts full bath* (temperature 110°F) twice weekly

4. *Cold friction bath* each afternoon

5. *Exercise* and abdominal massage. European specialists advocate hill climbing, bicycle riding, etc.

6. *Fasting*
   A. Water or fruit juices (4 to 5 days)
   B. Raw grated vegetables and fruits for the next week and a half. To this may be added olive oil, sour milk, bran, whole grains, molasses and fruit juices as you desire to taste.

FOOD CONTROL
FOR CONSTIPATION

Breakfast: stewed figs, prunes, on bran and milk

Morning break: fruit juices

Lunch: salad (chopped lettuce, onions, tomatoes,
grated carrots, spinach) with olive oil
and/or lemon juice

Afternoon break: Fruit juices or weak tea

Dinner: salad (same as for lunch)
fresh fruit, prunes, figs, raisins, yoghurt

Special Note: (a) develop regular bowel
evacuation habits. Respond immediately
when you get the urge. (b) Get rid of
all possible tensions and fears. Simply
walk away. Easier said than done? Have
you tried it?

EASY TREATMENT FOR
STOPPING DIARRHEA

Diarrhea is a watery stool that may or may not be accompanied by mucus and occurs frequently, or may be alternated with constipation. Diarrhea is a symptom. It is a signpost shouting—"There's trouble in the abdomen!" and too often this problem begins with excess starches in the diet, too much in the way of sugar, and too much meat. Allergies and drugs contribute to the problem and when the belly reacts in this manner it is Nature's protest against foreign and unacceptable material in the alimentary tract.

Most diarrhea occurs in the summer and may result from

neglect, improper eating habits, impure milk or water or even from nervous tension. Since diarrhea is Nature's way of expelling an irritating agent it should NOT be stopped! The problem lies in eliminating the cause. Where fever accompanies the problem rest in bed is very necessary. At this time eat no solids. For the most effective handling of the matter here are the—

STEPS TO TAKE:

1. FASTING—juice diet for three days. Drink copiously.

2. DAILY INTESTINAL LAVAGE or enema (salt water) each day of fasting. Water temperature: 75°.

3. COLD SECTIONAL ABLUTIONS consist of rubbing the skin briskly with cold water while standing in the tub nude. From bottom to top. Repeat every three hours. This stimulates the body and helps get rid of toxic waste from the body.

4. COLD HIP SITZ BATH (Review Figure 12) (40-50°F), ten minutes per session. Follow this with a friction rub of the entire body and extremities.

5. MASSAGE to thoroughly relax all muscles of the neck, back and abdominal muscles. End massage with digital pressure on the solar plexus area. Press deep for a five count. Release. Repeat at least four times.

6. POTATO DIET as strange as it may sound to us here in the U.S.A., works beautifully for diarrhea. I brought it from Europe. It's very simple to administer. Start after the third day of fasting with a baked potato (steamed or boiled with the skin on). *Use no salt!* Stay on this for three days.

STOMACH

DILATED STOMACH

When the stomach outlet refuses to operate to expel its contents—for any reason—and remains closed—food piles up in the stomach. Some digests. Some doesn't. The stomach sac begins to expand to hold the collecting contents. This act is called *dilation*. To cope with this problem I have found that that amazing water cure method called *"Neptune's Girdle"* is first choice in its care. The "girdle" is to be applied nightly. To this add a cold water spray on the abdomen. While this treatment is going on, eliminate all liquids by mouth. Solids such as cereals, meats and non-sugared fruits may be consumed in small amounts. In most part, avoid vegetables unless they have been macerated to mushlike consistency.

The *"Neptune's Girdle"* was a favorite treatment of Priessnitz, a European great. My granddad called this abdominal bandage "lieb-binde," and when you are looking for an effective method to treat the abdomen and its contents, and counteract excess gastric acidity, or even a fever, this is a method of choice.

How to Apply the Amazing "Neptune's Girdle"

Fold a cot-size bed sheet into fourths lengthwise. Soak three feet of one end of it in cold water. Start the wet end at the left side, just above the pelvis, and simply encircle the waist until all the dry sheeting has covered the wet section. If you don't want to go to that bother, saturate a large turkish towel after folding it into fourths. Saturate with cold water, suqeeze out the excess (50°-60°F cold water) and lay it over the abdomen while you are in a recumbent position in bed. Cover yourself with a plastic sheet and pull up the bed clothing. Go to sleep. In both methods, change the dressing as it becomes warm. As granddad said—"There's nothing better than lieb-binde when your belly is full and your brain congested with the problems of the day."

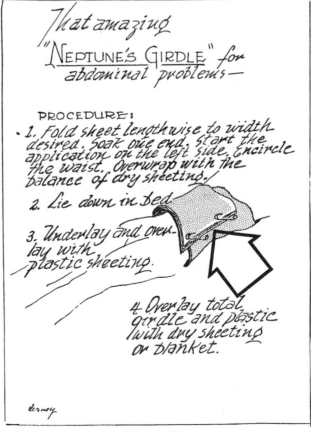

That amazing
"Neptune's Girdle" for
abdominal problems—

PROCEDURE:
1. Fold sheet lengthwise to width desired. Soak one end. Start the application on the left side. Encircle the waist. Overwrap with the balance of dry sheeting.

2. Lie down in bed.

3. Underlay and overlay with plastic sheeting.

4. Overlay total girdle and plastic with dry sheeting or blanket.

Figure 32

WHAT TO DO ABOUT
GASTRALGIA

Pain in the stomach is more often than not due to tension and is of "nervous" origin. Diet, and constitutional diseases, however, may cause it. In any case, if pain in your stomach is happening for the first time, or is *acute*, the object is to relieve pain and spasm and get the stomach wall relaxed. To accomplish this here are the—

STEPS TO TAKE:

1. HOT FOMENTATIONS An alternate method is to use a hot water bottle on the abdomen with a wet towel intervening. Place an additional hot water bottle, or hot wet fomentation, between the shoulder blades before bedtime. Maintain for 30 minutes to an hour. Be careful not to burn yourself with too much heat. As always, anoint yourself with oil before applying it.

2. HOT HALF SITZ BATH (105°F) for 30 minutes duration. (Figure 12).

3. HOT LIQUIDS ORALLY to be sipped slowly.

4. FOOD CONTROL must consist primarily of broths, cereals and fruits. Chew slowly. Masticate well.

HOW TO RELIEVE AND PREVENT
FLATULENCE *("Gas")*

**A Terrazo Floor Layer
Returns to Work After
Water Treatment**

I mention *flatulence* here, as a part of, or separate from dyspepsia, because it results from many conditions and yet need not be accompanied by heartburn and nausea as in dyspepsia.

Flatulence is an excessive accumulation of gas in the stomach and/or intestines. When gas collects in the stomach it may come out by belching. When it collects in the small and large intestine it may be expelled from the other end.

Ralph C.'s case was very pronounced. Any more gas and he would have floated away. Ralph's gas accumulated because of gulping air when he drank his vino. It came because he ate too much pasta. When he filled with gas, he couldn't stoop or bend over to do his job laying terrazo floors. He thought that he was going to have to retire. His son, Vittorio, got the same thing from drinking too much carbonated beverages and both protested that heredity was the cause of it all, that the discomfort they were having, the sensation of pressure, the fullness, the rumbling, the pressure on the heart, were normal to their family. They had to be convinced otherwise, that their flatulence was the result of over-eating, swallowing of air, gobbling food too fast, eating when exhausted, worried or angry. The moment Ralph and Vittorio conceded their problem might be something other than heredity, I took them off their heavy pastas, made them chew their foods, cut down smoking before meals, avoid excitement and live moderately, and a big change came. Along with this, I gave them instructions on the *cold sitz bath* which you, also, can use. Our biggest battle was with traditional eating and drinking habits. Once solved, the recovery for both was almost immediate. (For the Sitz Bath see Figure 12).

LACK OF GASTRIC JUICE
and What to Do About It

A great deal of stress is placed publicly on hyper-gastric acidity. But just as involved, perhaps even a greater problem, is the lack of gastric juice. To help yourself in this matter, the best hydrotherapy—in addition to regulating the diet and getting pepsin and hydrochloric acid in—is the cold or preferred ice pack on the abdomen. This should be applied ten minutes before a meal time. An abdominal Neptune's girdle (Review Figure 32) may be applied before meal time and before bedtime. Renew as it warms. At meal time precede all eating with a glassful of ice water. After that do not drink any other fluids with your meals. The ice water stimulates the gastric glands in the stomach wall. Digestive fluids begin to flow.

EXCESS GASTRIC ACIDITY
and How to Tone It Down

Very effective—in the hydrotherapy approach to this problem—is the use of the *Epsom salts bath*. Where hypergastric acidity exists, the salt absorbed by the body in the tub neutralizes the accumulation of acid waste. In utilizing this type of bath, use one and a half pounds of Epsom salts in a tub full of hot water (105°F) for ten minutes. DO NOT REMAIN IN THE TUB LONGER THAN TEN MINUTES. This type of treatment is excellent for rheumatic conditions as well as disorders of the stomach and bowel.

CAUTION:
DO NOT use this treatment
if you have a heart condition!

YOU CAN CONQUER
ACUTE GASTRITIS

Both hot and cold water treatments are used in the care of acute gastritis. For example, if there is vomiting, an *ice bag* is used over the stomach area and another placed between the shoulder blades. If there is pain, a *hot pack* should be used over the stomach. This pack should be renewed every ten minutes. Where the gastritis is the result of food poisoning, the stomach has to be emptied. Drinking tepid water with mustard in it will start vomiting to reduce the condition. Water therapy for gastritis from all causes is uniform.

Charlie G. had a lot of reasons for having his gastritis. He had violated all the health rules for years and expected to stay healthy and live forever. It just didn't work that way. In Charlie's case, it was too much alcohol and Mexican foods, too much tension and stress, too many zipper-upper drugs, improper diet and overeating, over-indulgence in everything, including girl friends. His belly was distended. He had a burning pain in his gut that extended up to his throat. He was constantly nauseated and vomiting. He was dizzy, had no desire to eat. His weight dropped. His tongue was coated and he had a breath that would stagger an elephant doctor. To conquer the problem, we set up the following program and it worked magic. I was delightfully surprised. So was he.

STEPS TO TAKE:

1. Alternate HOT/COLD HIP SITZ BATHS (Review Figure 12) Follow with cold sponging over entire body.

2. HOT FOMENTATIONS on abdomen to relieve discomfort AFTER eating.

3. EPSOM SALTS FULL BATH twice daily.

4. MASSAGE abdomen lightly.

5. FASTING for 24 hours. (Absolutely no solids, no milk) Juices (vegetable, fruit) only. Or, fast until the coating is gone from the tongue. After the second day, start on vegetable soup. You may drink lime blossom tea (your "Health Food" store has it). After the fourth day, eat fruit (apples, dates, prunes) salads (olive oil dressing or lemon juice), sour milk or yoghurt. AVOID all fried foods, pastries, white bread, sugar, condiments, tea, coffee "soft" drinks, over-indulgence in anything and everything.

6. FINGER-TIP PRESSURE ON THE SOLAR PLEXUS. While lying on your back, place finger tips of both hands into the pocket below the tip of the breastbone. Press deeply. Hold for a five count. Breath deeply. Release. Repeat for five minutes. Place ice pack on this area and go to sleep.

CHRONIC GASTRITIS

In *chronic gastritis* you will have no results unless you stick to the rules. What are the rules? (1) Give your stomach a rest. (2) Stop eating for 24 to 36 hours. (3) Avoid all alcoholic beverages, (4) Avoid spices, coffee, tea, cocoa, tobacco and rough bulky foodstuff.

STEPS TO TAKE:

1. WARM FULL BATH (Review Figure 16) to be taken immediately AFTER RISING FROM BED. (Water temp.: 95°-98°F) Ten minutes duration. Follow with a quick cold shower and brisk rubdown. A few seconds are all you need under the cold shower. It's a million-dollar tonic!

2. COLD ABDOMINAL COMPRESSES (Review Figure 1) are applied upon retiring for the night. Change as they warm. These packs may also be used during the day for pain relief.

3. HOT DRINKING WATER should be taken before breakfast. Two glasses full. Sip slowly.

HOW TO USE WATER AS A
CURE FOR INDIGESTION
(acute, chronic, nervous)

More often then not indigestion is caused by seven key factors. *Dyspepsia* is the technical handle given to this problem and its symptoms include heartburn, nausea, distress in the upper abdomen, gas and belching, bloating, all of them Nature's warning signals that something is direly wrong. Jason R. had all this and it occurred while eating and immediately after. The seven key factors that bring it on are: —(a) drinking fluids with meals, (b) inadequate or unwholesome diet (poorly cooked foods, high fat, gas-forming vegetables etc.), (c) eating too fast, (d) excessive or over-eating, (e) inadequate dentures and poor chewing habits, and, (f) eating while emotionally upset or tense, or (g) swallowing large amounts of air. Each contributes to the disaster of indigestion. Each provides a set of circumstances that the stomach is not prepared to handle. Taking drugs to mask or hide Nature's warning signals can prove disastrous, and for this reason, taking antiacid tablets and potions, etc. results in later complications.

With this in mind let's take a look at the program worked out for Jason R. Note how beautifully the relaxation bath works for you just as it did for him. Note how the fasting technique clears your eyes and brightens your day. Note how the simplified diet makes you feel like a million again. Stick to the rules of Food Control and you will have the sense of well-being that you've always wanted. It worked for Jason and it can work for you. His indigestion disappeared. There's been no report that he's had it since.

STEPS TO TAKE:

1. FULL RELAXATION BATH (Review Figure 16) water temperature 90°F. Hold this temperature in the bathtub for 30 minutes. No more. No less. Add some pine oil for fragrance.As the tensions relax within your body, the digestive mechanism will reorganize. Secretions will begin to flow normally. Peristalsis will be activated.

2. FASTING should continue for 10 to 14 days in all cases of indigestion or dyspepsia. Acute indigestion may require only a three-day fast. Chronics require 14. After the seventh day use the following—

FOOD CONTROL
FOR INDIGESTION

Breakfast: Fruit juice

Mid-morning: Fruit juice

Lunch: Lettuce salad with tomato, grated carrot
chopped onion and grated raw cabbage.
Serve with olive oil dressing or lemon
juice. Dessert: —baked apple

Mid-afternoon: Fruit juice or weak tea

Dinner: Fresh fruit, yoghurt, salad as at lunch.
To this diet you may add yeast or take
Vitamin B complex capsules.

Note: Take a 30-minute rest
AFTER EACH MEAL!
Do not eat if excited

3. INTESTINAL LAVAGE (enema—Review Figure 9). Administer daily to cleanse toxic bowel waste. As all this clears out, you will be relieved of foul breath and headaches that come with indigestion or the very changes that take place in fasting.

4. Alternate HOT/COLD SITZ HIP BATH (Review Figure 12). Alternate temperatures to be: —*hot* 115°F; *cold*, 65°F. Alternate at least twice and end with cold. Follow with—

5. COLD FRICTION Rub, or massage, on the abdomen. The purpose of these water procedures is to (a) reduce abdominal

congestion, (b) eliminate toxic waste, (c) strengthen and invigorate abdominal organs and their function, and, (d) help reestablish faulty blood circulation. *Massage* on the abdomen *should continue after the fasting period is completed.*

6. CORRECT POSTURE and habits have to be emphasized. Remember, no matter how effective the water therapy may be it cannot be of lasting value if you go right back to the bad habits that created your indigestion in the first place.

7. COLD WATER TREADING (Review Figure 5) Here's what Margaret says about her variation of water treading:—

> *"I stand in a tub full of warm water in the nude. Under the cold water faucet I douse a cold towel, squeeze it, and then start rubbing myself vigorously from the feet up. I work up toward the heart from the extremities. I never feel the cold this way. The friction starts me glowing. My tensions evaporate! I pass gas. My bowels move and I come out of the bathroom feeling like a million. I'm ready to handle my big family once more."*

One more water therapy "trick" you can use to step up your health program even faster is to sit in cold, rather than warm, water. Do this for five minutes. Rub down briskly and you're ready for anything.

8. HOT COMPRESSES (Review Figure 1) to the sides of the neck (over the vagus nerve) and over the solar plexus area will help neutralize the inflammatory situation in the digestive tract. This treatment is aided and abetted by—

9. COLD COMPRESSES placed simultaneously over the thoracic (upper and middle back) at least once daily for 30 minutes per session.

10. DIETARY CONTROLS as indicated in "Fasting" segment. Maintain a "balanced diet." Eat slowly! Chew thoroughly. No matter what the rush may be refuse to gobble and run. Control the circumstances and environment around you as much as possible. Avoid everything unpleasant. Walk away from places and people who are unpleasant during meal times.

11. SOCIALLY avoid gossip, sarcasm and everything that will keep you emotionally involved.

12. PLENTY OF REST. Make a point of scheduling and controlling your sleep routine. Permit no one to interfere with it. Guard your health rights jealously. Your biggest responsibility is to yourself and your personal health. Everything else comes second.

HOW TO STOP NAUSEA
AND FEEL GOOD AGAIN

Nausea is the desire to vomit. Sometimes you vomit. Sometimes you don't, but you still "feel like it." Nausea may stem from eye problems, balance center insecurity in the ear or brain, odors, hysterical conditions, sea or air sickness, and/or pregnancy. It may come with gall bladder problems, heights, car sickness. No matter what the cause one of the more effective measures I have found to cope with it is water therapy! Here are the—

STEPS TO TAKE:

1. ICE PACK at the base of the skull and neck and another over the solar plexus area. *Time*: 30 minutes.

2. MASSAGE the muscles of the back with special attention given to the painful areas that may be noted along the spinal column from the neck to the tailbone.

STEPS TO TAKE IN GETTING
RID OF ULCERS
(gastric and duodenal)

The job of the stomach is to manufacture gastric juices to

digest foods entering it. Excess of such acid may go further than just breaking down foodstuffs for general metabolism. It may also eat a hole in the lining of the stomach. This is an *ulcer*. The stomach actually eats itself. It may occur at the point where the stomach empties into the small intestine. This is called the duodenum. When you are tense, worried or anxious it starts up. The problem happens most often in men between the ages of 20 and 40. It may occur, however, in women after menopause.

Sarah J. had full-blown ulcers. Sarah is a business executive, a driver. She never stops going. Even in her few hours of sleep she twitches and thrashes in bed. The problem that brought her to my office was the burning or gnawing pain she had AFTER meals. She had hunger pains at night and would get out of bed to take an alkalizer. Sometimes the discomfort was relieved by vomiting, sometimes by milk or medication. Then it got worse. The program we worked out for Sarah was instrumental in getting her back on the job. Within a week's time, she reported big improvement by using the following techniques:—

STEPS TO TAKE:

1. GET RID OF THE SOURCE OF TENSION! In Sarah's case, it was two men on the staff who were trying to take her job away from her. I didn't suggest that she bump them off but I did discuss the women's equal rights law and she followed through. Other tensions may begin at home and the point is that you have to learn to relax under any and all circumstances. To help you relax here's the—

2. RELAXING FULL BATH (Review Figure 16) once daily 30 to 60 minutes per day just before going to bed. Alternate with hot/cold hip sitz baths each day.

3. POSTURAL IMPROVEMENT is vital. Stand erect! In this position the pressure is taken off your stomach.

4. COLD SECTIONAL ABLUTIONS, three or four times daily with gentle but brisk friction rub of the entire body.

5. RECTAL ENEMAS with nutrients where food cannot be taken by mouth. Continue intestinal lavages (enemas) until the symptoms subside. Here now are some key factors:—

WHERE THE FOLLOWING CONDITIONS ARE PRESENT

(A) *Hemorrhaging in the stomach*. Use *hot* rectal enemas four times daily. Maintain water temperature at 110° to 115°F.

(B) *Abdominal stomach pain*. May be handled with hot packs over the belly. Maintain water temperature at 120°F. Also place hot packs between the shoulder blades. With this excellent procedure the pain diminishes. The wild motility of the stomach slows down. Excess gastric acidity decreases. The relief is almost dramatic. *Alternate this* with a Scotch Douche or hot spray over the abdomen, followed by a quick cold shower. This is especially effective where the pain does not diminish from heat therapy alone.

(C) *Where there is anemia* associated with gastric ulceration, the best water therapy approach is the use of cold sectional ablutions. Briskly rub the body with cold water at least twice daily for three weeks. Twice weekly thereafter.

GALL BLADDER AND LIVER

Biliousness
Cholecystitis
Gall stones
Jaundice

REVITALIZING THAT AILING GALL BLADDER
AND STOPPING BILIOUSNESS

When Karen F. came into the office, her complaint was that she was *bilious*. That's a dirty word but sure enough she was. Biliousness is a symptom of liver disorder. She told me that she was constipated, vomited up bile, had headaches and didn't have any appetite. The answer to Karen's problem was in the following program . . . and her symptoms disappeared one by one.

STEPS TO TAKE:

1. COLD ABDOMINAL COMPRESSES (Review Figure 1) nightly if the biliousness is chronic. In acute cases use—

2. ALTERNATE HOT/COLD COMPRESSES on the abdomen. Hot water application for one minute; five minutes cold. Continue this process for two hours.

3. INTESTINAL LAVAGE (Review Figure 9) twice daily Water temperature at 75° to 80°F. Add one tablespoonful of salt to each quart of water used.

4. DIETARY CONTROLS must consist of a very light diet (soup, broth, fish). AVOID overeating! DO NOT eat meat or other fatty substances. DO NOT eat eggs. DO NOT drink anything alcoholic, tea or coffee.

5. EXERCISE regularly. Keep active with long brisk walks, bicycle riding, running in place, etc.

HOW TO RELIEVE CHOLECYSTITIS
VIA NATURE'S WAY

Cholecystitis means inflammation of the gall bladder. The gall bladder is a sac about the length of your thumb. It's a stretchable sac that hangs down into the abdomen from the underside of the liver. In general, it's a storehouse for bile. The liver manufactures about a quart of bile per day, and as the temporary storage place for bile, empties it into the small intestine when necessary. Digestion, without bile, is incomplete. Where constipation and gastritis exist there is usually inflammation in the gall bladder. There may also be stones in the sac, but they don't necessarily spell out trouble unless one of them gets in an awkward position in the gall duct.

Although all signs and symptoms of gall bladder problems don't always appear in apple-pie order, they were par for the course for Marjorie M. She had severe colicky pain in her abdomen, vomiting, nausea, feeling of fullness after eating, pressure below the breastbone, heartburn, gas, and pains that were more severe at night than during the day. Sometimes her pain radiated up between her shoulder blades. Sometimes the pain was under the right shoulder blade, sometimes down the right arm.

Marjorie's husband dug me out of bed at three o'clock in the morning to treat her problem. Treating Marjorie was like treating a brick wall. She didn't listen, refused to cooperate, just cried and complained. She'd been to a lot of doctors of other professions and cried and complained for their benefit as well. Because she didn't stick to the rules, she got fatter and fatter, ate constantly of foods made with white flour and white sugar, never ate fruits or vegetables, refused to exercise, was constipated and took every nostrum she could get from the druggist's shelf. Her husband tried to get her to stop wailing in my office so that I could discuss what she could to to help herself or she was going to be dead. He didn't get anywhere. Then I saw a wondrous thing happen. That poor little henpecked man lct loose with a slap in the face that made her jowls jump. Her mouth popped open in surprise. So did her eyes. Then her mouth shut and she was silent. She listened. It was our first big breakthrough!

STEPS TO TAKE:

1. FASTING on water and fruit and vegetable juices. *Note:*

The length of the fast depends on the duration of the gall bladder or liver problem. For best results count on at least three weeks of fasting. Every fourth day eat some raw fruits, raw salads, steamed vegetables. Add small amounts of protein. Add very little starch or fat to your diet. If progress is favorable, allow two weeks before starting another fast. For ten days eat raw fruit, raw salad and steamed vegetables. The balance of four days you can add poached eggs, cheese, nuts, wholewheat toast. You will begin to notice a definite weight loss.

2. INTESTINAL LAVAGE (enema) daily (85°F) during fasting. Discontinue all enemas the moment fasting stops!

3. COLD HIP SITZ BATH and cold friction rub each morning. As an interesting note on Marjorie M., I was entering her home on a house call when I heard her wailing from the bathroom. I heard her husband calmly tell her to get into the cold water tub or he was going to spank her, that she had already lost 60 pounds of blubber, that she had improved 1,000 percent and if she kept at it she would look just as she did the day they were married. It was the best psychology I've ever heard. I let myself out unannounced. They never knew I was there. Why should I tell them? Everything was going great!

4. HOT COMPRESSES OR FOMENTS (Review Figures 1 and 31) if there is any local abdominal pain. Treat daily for a week. Then alternate hot/cold for a week thereafter. Fifteen minutes for each for one hour. Follow promptly with—

5. MASSAGE of the abdomen, upper and lower back. Massage the abdomen ONLY after one week of back massage. Give special attention to the painful areas between the shoulder blades. Massage them until the pain dissipates and is gone.

6. EXERCISE PROGRAM should begin immediately to help burn up the calories. Supplement exercise with deep breathing. To help in her program, Marjorie joined a "health studio." You'll never believe it but she lost 98 pounds! And it all began with her gall bladder and a thing called *cholecystitis*.

7. FLUIDS, water and fruit and vegetable juices copiously.

GALL STONES
and How Hydrotherapy Is the Treatment of Choice

Gall stones are more apt to occur in women than in men. They are more apt to occur in the obese or pregnant woman. Nobody knows exactly why a gall stone happens yet we do know that the menstrual cycle plays some role in its formation. Most of the time folks don't even know they have "stones." But when a stone IS actively causing nausea, vomiting and cramps (especially after a big meal) you know it! If the pain gets worse, it may radiate to the right scapula and shoulder. Maybe a slight fever. Sometimes a passing jaundice (yellow skin). In gall stone problems, the "attack" stops rather abruptly after intense pain. Why? Usually the stone has dropped back down into the gall bladder sac. But the interim period—up to two hours of abdominal stress—marks a kind of hell all its own. To prevent it—(a) *reduce weight,* (2) *control your diet* (little or no fat), high protein, high carbohydrates and limited calories, (3) *supplement your diet* with Vitamins A, D, and K. But when the pain comes the treatment of choice is water therapy. Here's how to do it: —

STEPS TO TAKE:

1. ICE PACK to be placed between the shoulder blades.

2. HOT HALF BATHS are the most advantageous for acute "attacks" of gall stones. Start the water temperature at 100°F as you sit in the tub. Add hot water gradually until it is 105°F. *Time:* ten minutes ONLY. End the treatment with a quick cold shower and brisk rubdown with a rough towel.

ALTERNATE TREATMENT
FOR GALL STONES

HOT FOMENTS to be used on alternate days with the hot half baths. Place foment on the abdomen. *Time:* five minutes. Alternate with COLD FOMENTS. Treatment time: two minutes.

Repeat the alternations for two hours or until the symptoms are relieved.

Reminder: **always anoint the abdomen with**
olive oil before applying the hot foment.

3. HOT WATER ENEMA (as hot as you can stand) to relieve abdominal spasms. Apply while lying on your back on the bathroom floor. Retain the fluid as long as you can hold it. Then get up on the stool and evacuate.

4. COLD COMPRESSES on the abdomen (Review Figure 1) before bedtime each evening. Time: 1 hour. Renew as it warms.

YELLOW JAUNDICE
. . . AND WHAT TO DO ABOUT IT

Jaundice is a yellowing of the skin and of the whites of the eyes due to possible changes in the liver or obstruction of the bile in its flow to the small intestine. When cut off by spasm, stones, or pressure, the bile backs up into the blood stream and is carried throughout the body. The urine gets dark, the feces gets a claylike color, there's a loss of appetite and a feeling of lassitude. Sometimes the skin itches for no apparent reason. Your heart may start beating like sixty and the first thing to do is see your doctor about the cause. After that, there is a hydrotherapy method you can use to get rid of that unsightly skin discoloration and physical discomfort.

STEPS TO TAKE:

1. Alternate HOT/COLD COMPRESSES to the abdomen. Maintain hot compreses for one minute at 120°F. Alternate with cold compresses at 60°F for five minutes. Continue for one hour

or at least ten repetitions. Repeat the procedure at six-hour intervals.

2. HOT WATER ENEMA three times daily while lying on your back on the bathroom floor. (Water temperature: 105°F)

3. LIQUIDS COPIOUSLY: Water, fruit and vegetable juices, preferably hot.

Note: after the acute attack subsides, use a cold compress on the abdomen nightly for one week. Continue this process every fourth week for six months.

4. WARM FULL RELAXATION BATHS are excellent if you are itching with your jaundice. Remain submerged for five minutes. Start tub at 100°F. Gradually add hot water to 105°F. Keep a cold wet turban (a wet towel or ice bag) on your head. Renew it as it warms. Complete your treatment with a fast cold shower, rub down with a coarse dry towel and go to bed. Each day you will be less and less discolored if your waste outlets begin to work properly once more. You'll simply wonder where the yellow went.

water
treatment
for the
LOWER
EXTREMITIES

chapter

8

Subjects covered

Arthritis
Cold Feet
Rheumatism
Sciatica
Sprains and strains
Edema (swelling)
Varicose veins

ARTHRITIS AND
NATURE'S BEST HEALERS

The word *arthritis,* like a lot of other medical words, is a catch-all. As a physical condition it means inflammation of a joint. As a word, it is what you call a problem in or around a joint when you can't specifically identify or name it. There's no one kind of arthritis. Arthritis may come from infectious disease or follow a fever. It may result from degenerate diseases. It may come as the result of the nervous system being involved. It may come about because of disturbances in body metabolism such as gout. But there is one thing that almost all arthritics have in common. That's discomfort and hurt, and heat still remains one of the best therapies for the chronic case of this "dread disease." Hot water therapy, followed by cold water, is the method of choice. If you have had arthritis in the past—or have it in the present—you will remember how badly you wanted relief. Well there is relief . . . and there are no drugs involved. No matter what the cause, here's what to do for an inflamed joint:—

STEPS TO TAKE:

ACUTE JOINT PROBLEMS

1. HOT COMPRESSES (Review Figure 1) applied every 15 minutes for an hour. Keep the following key in mind:—

As quickly as joint discomfort or pain subsides—under hot applications—give that joint cold affusions immediately!

(*Affusion*-rubbing the skin briskly with hands full of cold water). Dry the part and keep it warm. A knee, for example, may be kept warm with the sleeve cut from an old sweater. Simply pull it up over your knee. Maintaining warmth in an arthritic joint is worth a million dollars in saved pains in the future.

CHRONIC JOINT PROBLEMS

STEPS TO TAKE:

1. HOT AIR AND STEAM BATHS are most effective for chronic joint problems. Treatment time is never longer than two hours. Hot air, or steam, stimulates local tissues and steps up the elimination of toxic waste. Absorption of toxic waste from in and

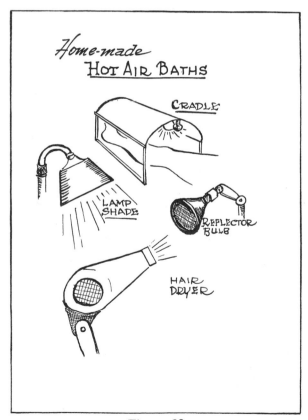

Figure 33

around the joint is produced within 20 minutes. At this point, relaxation in surrounding tissues takes place. Always follow heat therapy on the extremities with cold ablutions (pour cold water on them or spray them as did the great German hydrotherapist, Kneipp, with a watering can. During treatment, keep the part moving. Start exercising that joint immediately when the tissue becomes warm. Move it! Don't baby it! Homemade warming devices such as those illustrated in Figure 33 may be used.

HOW TO CURE
COLD FEET OVERNIGHT

Dancer Effectively Treats
Cold Feet Treading Water

Every now and again the problem of "cold feet" pops up. When this happens folks want to know—"What can I do for it?" Coldness in the extremities can have complicated causes. It may be caused by hardening of the arteries, from nervous excitement or even from anemia. It may stem from faulty diet or inadequate bowel movement.

In Jean Marie's case it was caused by pressure on her extremities and waist. Jean's a dancer. After a number of years as a chorus girl in a Las Vegas casino, she opened her own dancing school. Most of her time was spent in teaching. Most of the time she had on her tights. As time went along she began to complain of cold feet. She couldn't understand why her extremities felt like ice even when she was so active. And how come, she wanted to know, when she was on vacation in Florida and paddling in the ocean, her feet WERE NOT cold? To answer that question, I examined her and found a healthy young woman. Everything A-OK. Then why the cold feet? Her question about not having cold feet at the seashore was my first clue. As far as Jean Marie was concerned, it was water therapy—unconsciously administered—that did the trick. But even more then that was the fact she was not wearing those tight tights. They were cutting off her circulation as effectively as a tourniquet. I called this to her attention and she said she could get rid of the tights but she couldn't be running down to Miami Beach every weekend for a dose of sea water on her legs and feet. I told her she could get the same results in a bathtub at home! How? Treading water and here's how it's done:—

STEPS TO TAKE:

1. WATER TREADING (Review Figure 5). With water mid-calf-high, pace back and forth in cold water until your feet experience a flush of warmth. This is your cue to step out of the tub, wipe your feet briskly with a coarse towel and get into warm footgear if you are going to remain out of bed. *Note*: Here's the trick:—*If you go to bed, go to bed with your feet wet!*

Alternates to the
above procedure:

A. Walking barefoot in the dewy grass.
B. The Kneipp procedure in which—while sitting on the edge of the bathtub—simply spray your extremities with a watering can, or a bathtub spray.

2. COLD HIP SITZ BATH (Review Figure 12) nightly before bedtime. Treatment *time*: five minutes. Temperature: 65°F and into bed after a brisk rubdown with a coarse towel. My grandfather used this method and never once—although he lived past 80—did he complain of cold feet.

> *A recommended additive: Also place a cold compress on the low back and tailbone. Keep changing it as it warms. It will make you feel wonderful all over.*

INFECTIONS

The year was 1920. I jumped off the back of the horse-drawn ice wagon where I was snitching a piece of ice. My bare feet didn't hit the pavement direct. One foot came down on a board full of nails lying in the street. One of the spikes went up through my foot between the metatarsal bones. I sat down in the middle of the street, took a big gulp, and pried the board off. The entire leg became involved. The doctor took one look and shook his head and said—"The leg must go!" My mother burst out crying. "Amputation is necessary," he insisted.

"Nein," said my grandfather who was visiting us from Michigan. "I fix." He did. He took me home, sat me in the sunny back yard, placed my foot and leg in a bucket of cold water. It was a big wooden bucket filled to the brim. As the sun warmed the water, he ladled it out and poured cold water in. He repeated this for four days for five hours each day. "Das iss goot," said my grandfather in mollifying my mother. "All will be well." and it was.

On the fourth day, the foot opened. Corruption came rolling out in cream-colored clouds. Grandpa rinsed the leg off and laid me in the sun. Every day I had the same kind of warm air bath. Healing began. Maybe I was lucky. Maybe it was another miracle in water therapy, but I still have my legs today.

In addition to the cold tub bath you can use contrast baths for lower extremity infections, saline baths, cold compresses and spraying techniques. Here are the—

STEPS TO TAKE:

1. COLD SPIRAL COMPRESS. To do this fold a turkish towel lengthwise into thirds. Saturate with cold water. Wrap arm and hand or foot and leg from the distal tip upwards. Re-apply as it warms. As the procedure continues, you will note pulsation from the infection has begun to subside. Redness will disappear. Swelling departs. *Note*: at no time use heat on a new infection. As an alternate to this method, wrap the extremity and douse ice water on it even while remembering always to permit the warming process to take place.

2. SCOTCH DOUCHE (spray technique) (Review Figure 7). The moment an infection begins utilize the magic of water therapy. While sitting on the edge of the tub, spray the offended extremity from top to bottom. Make slow excursions up and down. Keep the process going until a feeling of coldness permeates your fingers, hand, and arm. It may even feel somewhat numb. When the spraying is discontinued a reaction sets in. The extremity becomes red and warm. With that new and natural heat suffusing your extremity, wrap the part with dry toweling. Get into bed or just sit down and rest. Repeat three times daily for best results. When water treatment is applied healing is always clean, neat, and uninvolved. There is little or no scar tissue.

At-a-Glance Information

Additional Health Problems
You Can Treat with

SCOTCH DOUCHE

Bladder problems   Hemorrhoids
High Blood Pressure   Sprains/Strains
Constipation   Varicose veins

How and where:

Cold sprays (to quell local inflammation or irritation such as varicose veins or bites.

Tepid sprays on the spine and used for neurasthenia and other nerve conditions.

Cold sprays on the spine for hemorrhoids, high blood pressure, bladder conditions and constipation.

---

3. CONTRAST BATHS can be administered by utilizing two buckets. One bucket for cold water (65°F). One for warm

water at 105°-110°F. Place feet in hot water for three minutes. Dip into cold water for 30 seconds. Back into the hot water for three minutes and end with cold. What have you done? You have first dilated the blood vessels with heat and then made them contract under the influence of cold. In ending with cold therapy you set the physiological stage for a series of reflex actions. The cold feeling in your extremities begins to disappear. They glow and it's a comforting feeling of well-being. The body feels it also. The mind feels it! As one of my lady patients said to me—"Fix my cold feet and you'll fix my personality!"

4. SALINE FOOT BATH. To a bucket of warm water (105°F), add a handful of table salt. Mix until dissolved. Add feet. Soak for 20 minutes. With one foot remaining in the pail, start scrubbing the other foot with a soft brush. This will not only innervate the circulation, but will help you get rid of corns, calluses, dryness of skin and other foot discomforts. If the water cools add more hot water. Treat each foot to this happiness and end the scrubbing with a quick dip into the cold water bucket. Just in and out. Rub briskly with a dry coarse towel. *Don't leave your feet exposed* after the hot salt bath if you would take full advantage of the physiological reaction that follows. Don shoes and stockings immediately!

HOW TO CONTROL
RHEUMATIC PAIN

Rheumatism is a non-health problem with fever, pain, inflammation and swelling in or near a bony joint. Soft tissues, such as the muscles, ligaments, tendons and connective tissue of all kinds, may all become involved. Rheumatism may be known by the name of *lumbago* when it occurs in the back, as *torticollis* when you get it in the neck, as *charley horse* when it occurs in the legs and thighs.

When Casey P. developed his rheumatism, it laid him up. He couldn't work. His joints were inflamed, swollen and sore.

He had a fever that went as high as 103°F and then dropped to 97.8°F. The whole problem came on abruptly. Large joints (Knees, ankles, elbows, wrists) got red, swollen and extremely tender to touch. He had a sore throat and felt chilly all the time. He perspired like mad and, on testing, his sweat showed an acid reaction. His face was red, his tongue heavily coated, his bowels were not moving and he was in total misery. For Casey, I set up the following program. Within two weeks, pain, stiffness, and redness had gone. No deformities. Happily his heart valves were uninvolved. Usually the outcome is unfavorable in most cases of rheumatism. In Casey's case, the batting average was very good. If you would accomplish the same success, here are the—

STEPS TO TAKE:

1. COMPLETE BED REST in a ventilated room free of drafts. For greatest ease in bed, sleep between blankets rather then sheets. They are softer to those aching joints.

2. CONTRAST BATHS (Scotch Douche) (See Figure 15). Alternately spray joints with hot and cold water (hands, feet, ankles, wrist, elbows, knees). While sitting nude on the edge of the bathtub, attach the rubber spray hose to the bathtub faucet. Spray hot water (110°F) against the aching joint for *one minute*. Follow immediately with cold spray for 30 seconds. Maintain hot/cold on the aching joint until the pain dulls away. Then go to the next joint. Spray technique may be used on other parts of the body (if the rheumatism "spreads). Three mornings a week, spray the lower extremities and buttocks. On alternate nights, spray the back and shoulders. One minute is enough treatment time for each joint.

3. COLD SPIRAL WRAP (including surrounding muscles) (Review Figure 4 for technique). Fold a turkish towel lengthwise in thirds. Saturate with cold water (60°F) and spiral up the ex- tremity (hand or foot). Permit wrap to warm. Remove, re- saturate, wring and re-apply for at least an hour session, three

times daily or until the pain subsides. Placing the wrapped part in a plastic dry cleaning bag will help to keep the spiral wrap from getting everything else wet. It will also maintain cold.

4. "X" WRAP COLD COMPRESS (Review Figure 18). Apply the "X" wrap, twice weekly for six weeks, over the thorax and abdomen for general revitalization. It will not only improve your sleep, but step up better body metabolism. I admit that a certain amount of discomfort comes with water therapy. Surely, it's inconvenient. But it gets results! And that's what you're after! Note the discomfort diminish. Note the follow-up reaction of pleasurable warmth and relaxation. As an alternate to the "X" wrap, you can use the *Hot Full Bath,* or the *Rise-and-Fall-Bath.* (See Figure 34.)

5. DIETARY CONTROLS:
   A. Diluted fruit juices, glassful on the half hour.
   B. No pastries, sugars, meats. Stick to vegetables and fruits . . . two-day diet.

6. HABITS:
   A. Keep bowels and kidneys cleaned out.
   B. Take daily walks
   C. Air bathing[1] (nude) for one hour per day.
   D. Rest.

SCIATICA
. . . and What to Do About It

The sciatic nerve is the longest nerve you have. It exits from the spinal column in the low back and sends branches all the way to the foot. The longer the inflammation lasts in the sciatic nerve,

---

[1]*Air Bathing* is the total exposure of the nude body while going through light calisthenics and breathing rhythmically to the tempo of your exercise. One hour per day, anywhere within the range of your modesty. Follow your air bath with a "friction-body-rub." Mittens or a coarse towel will do. Rub from foot to head.

the more extremity parts become involved. How quickly they get involved depends on the cause. Inflammation and pain in this giant nerve may begin with a direct blow. It may come from the position of a foetus in the pelvis pressing against it, from infections, from other physical or chemical changes in the body. It may be referred from some other body part. For example, Jack D. hit the bottle quite a bit. He ate very little. Result: Vitamin B deficiency and sciatic nerve irritation. Tommy F. got his from a sacro-iliac joint separation in a football game. Marteen G. had an ulcer on her anus that started it off. Sciatic inflammation may come from a fall, a twist, or sometimes what appears to be nothing at all.

As far as the pain is concerned, sciatica may start as a dull gnawing ache in the leg. It may begin in the buttock. It may extend as far as the heel of the foot. Your only clue may be a feeling of numbness along the outside of the foot. When there's a sharp stabbing pain up the thigh, it's usually a sign that the cause lies in the spinal bones or disc areas. If a bowel movement or sneeze starts the pain, it's the nerve roots involved at the spinal cord. It's all very complex and quite often it's necessary to see your doctor. In all cases, however, you can give yourself a great deal of relief through the suggested water therapies that follow. Here are the—

STEPS TO TAKE:

1. HALF HIP SITZ BATH (Review Figure 12). Alternate days for three weeks using a neutral water temperature (90°F). Sit down in two inches of tepid water in the tub. Turn the cold water on. Let it run till the water temperature drops to 60°F. Turn the water off. Sit only as long as the water gets as high as your umbilicus. The next day, for one minute after the water height gets to this point. The third day, hold for three minutes. *Note: If you have a heart condition do NOT use this method!*

2. SCOTCH DOUCHE (cold water, 60°F).

Morning: spray *ONLY the low back and extremities* while standing in the bathtub nude. Treatment time: 30-40 seconds. Or, hold the cold spray on the sore spots as long as you can stand it. When the pain dulls out, stop the treatment. That's it! Dry yourself briskly. Don warm clothing and go about your regular business.

Evening: On alternate evenings, for two weeks, spray *the upper back*. Rub briskly and go to bed. Wrap warmly. Sleep well. If the leg or thigh pain persists turn the full force of the spray on the sore spot for 20 seconds only.

3. RISING-AND-FALLING BATH

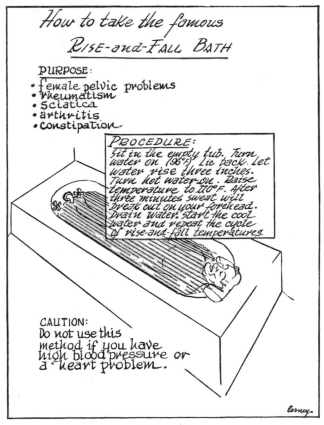

How to take the famous RISE-and-FALL BATH

PURPOSE:
- female pelvic problems
- rheumatism
- sciatica
- arthritis
- constipation

PROCEDURE:
Sit in the empty tub. Turn water on (98°F.) Lie back. Let water rise three inches. Turn hot water on. Raise temperature to 110°F. After three minutes sweat will break out on your forehead. Drain water. Start the cool water and repeat the cycle of rise-and-fall temperatures.

CAUTION:
Do not use this method if you have high blood pressure or a heart problem.

Figure 34

INSTANT RELIEF FOR SPRAINED ANKLE

Maybe you've never sprained an ankle. But when it happens, you have to know what to do to prevent all the repercussions that may follow. Such as? Swelling, black-and-blueness because blood vessels are torn, pain and discomfort and follow-ups. Locate the exact spot that hurts. This will identify the ligament or ligaments involved. The secret here is immediate care. If you are outdoors away from civilization, but near a creek, stream, or lake, promptly dunk your foot. Cold is the immediate objective followed by getting back into your shoe. Lace the shoe tightly and walk! Where more facilities are available, use the following:—

STEPS TO TAKE:

1. COLD WATER SPIRAL WRAP (Review Figure 4)

Fill a bucket with cold water. Dump in a trayful of ice cubes. Now fold a large turkish towel in thirds lengthwise. Dunk it into the cold water. Squeeze. Spirally wrap from foot to knee. The secret here is DO NOT REMOVE THE WRAP!. Over the area of pain, and over the wet towel, place an ice bag. Elevate the foot. *Treatment time:* one hour every six hours. After the 12-hour period, hot compresses may begin. By this time the small blood vessels have stopped bleeding. Swelling recedes. The pain is gone.

2. DIRECT ICE THERAPY

Place the offended extremity immediately into an icewater bath, an ice pack, or rub the part with an ice cube. This excellent procedure not only relieves pain but diminishes the problem of broken vessels and hastens healing.

3. COTTON ELASTIC OR ADHESIVE TAPE SECURITY WRAPS

HOW TO COPE WITH
SWOLLEN FEET

Si G. had had swollen legs and feet for as far back as he could remember. Si is a house painter. He has spent a lifetime up and down ladders and, over the years, the pressure of rungs in the arch of his foot cut off circulation. As a result, he developed varicose vains and a couple of fat legs. He said he felt as if he was walking on posts. The water therapy program for him proved effective. Today, his feet are no longer swollen. He wears his shoes in comfort and his job has become less toil and more fun.

STEPS TO TAKE:

1. ALTERNATE CONTRAST FOOT BATHS. Fill two buckets, one with hot water (115°F). The other with cold (60°F). As you sit in your favorite chair, dunk both feet into the hot water for three minutes. Then 30 seconds in the cold. Alternate the procedure at least four times. Don warm footgear and move around. Or, go to bed, wrap warmly, and sleep.

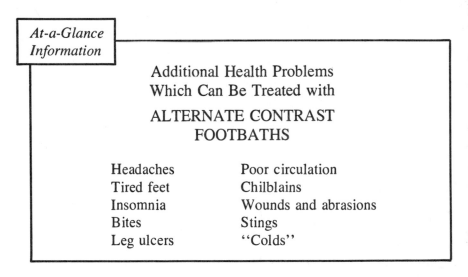

At-a-Glance
Information

Additional Health Problems
Which Can Be Treated with

ALTERNATE CONTRAST
FOOTBATHS

Headaches	Poor circulation
Tired feet	Chilblains
Insomnia	Wounds and abrasions
Bites	Stings
Leg ulcers	"Colds"

2. SCOTCH DOUCHE: Sit on the edge of the bathtub and spray your extremities with tepid water, from the thighs down. Do this every day for a month and twice weekly thereafter. You will find this not only comforting but it will make you drowsy. End with cold but DO NOT DRY YOUR FEET if you are going to bed immediately. Wrap yourself warmly with blankets and sleep.

3. COLD COMPRESS. Apply large folded turkish towel-

ing (cold water 60°F) over the point of pain. . This may be alternated with the spiral wrap from toe to knee. Re-apply both as they get warm. *Time:* 1 hour.

4. TAKE A DIURETIC: Activating the kidneys is always of value where the legs and feet are swollen. The more the kidneys function, the more excess water is dumped from the system. For this purpose I suggest buchu and juniper berries, crushed and steeped in boiling water. Drink a glassful of the tea twice daily. *Procedure:* Boil water in a saucepan. Crush the berries. Drop them into the boiling water. Turn off the heat. Let the berries steep. Then cool. Keep the mixture in the refrigerator. (Buchu and juniper berries are obtainable at your health food store).

VARICOSE VEINS
and How to Subdue Them

Pregnancy, occupation, obesity, dietary deficiencies, heredity, etc. are all factors contributing to varicose veins. A varicose vein is a vessel whose wall has developed a weak area in it and bulged. You have probably seen some around. One case I will never forget was Shean K! He was one of my overweight, overzealous, overage football players. He had a thing about proving to his little son that Dad was still able to play as he had back in college. Shean wanted his kid to look up to him. There's nothing wrong with that but the problem with Shean was that he wouldn't stick to the rules.

So during one of our away games, 38-year-old Shean got cleated in the leg. A varicose vein broke. Bleeding was profuse. He had to be hospitalized. When he was released the bleeding was stopped but an ulcer had begun. The leg swelled. He had pain in his foot and ankle. Despite being informed not to return to football, he returned to the clubhouse and girded for battle. The vessel broke again. Back he went to the hospital for venous repair.

There are a lot of folks just as stubborn about their feet and legs and sooner or later complications arise. If you have varicosities, the following water therapy procedures can be of great value to you in bringing comfort and relief. They won't get rid of the varicose veins, but you will be feeling better because circulation has been improved. If, in some emergency situation, you break a vein, DO NOT apply a tourniquet. Put your finger right into the spot. Press. Hold. Apply a clean dressing as it stops and get to your doctor. I repeat DO NOT USE A TOURNIQUET. Don't walk for at least 12 hours. Elevate legs and feet above heart level. For lesser varicosities here's the process to use:—

STEPS TO TAKE:

1. COLD HALF HIP SITZ BATH (Review Figure 12) to be used three times weekly before bedtime. While water is running into the tub undress. Keep your upper half warm with a sweater. Have a blanket ready for when you exit to bed. Sit down in the water. Remain 30 seconds. Get up. Do NOT dry yourself. Instead, wrap the blanket around you and rush to bed. Cover warmly. Remain one hour, after which time you get up, dress warmly and move around actively.

2. SCOTCH DOUCHE (Review Figure 15) Cold back and hip sprays may be used on alternate nights, or, in conjunction with the hip-sitz baths, because of their powerful stimulative effect. In dealing with varicose veins, take this invigorating cold shower immediately each morning upon getting out of bed.

3. COLD SPIRAL LEG WRAP (Review Figure 4). Spiral the cold pack from foot to knee. Place wraps on *both* legs although only one may be currently involved; with your bed previously prepared with plastic sheeting to keep from saturating the bed. Wrap yourself warmly. Leave the wraps as they are. If you are still awake after an hour, remove the wrap. Throw it on the floor. Go to sleep. If you do fall asleep, simply leave it on until you awaken. Then throw it off on the floor and go to sleep again.

4. WATER TREADING (Review Figure 5)

water
treatment
for the
SKIN

---

chapter
9

Subjects covered:

Eczema
Fevers
Prostration
Sunstroke

THE NEW
COLD WATER TECHNIQUE
FOR ACUTE ECZEMA

STEPS TO TAKE:

1. COLD COMPRESSES OR COLD WET FOMENT (Review Figures 1 and 6). Wrap the involved parts with thick soft cloth. Moisten the cloth with COLD water (55°-60°F) every 15 to 30 minutes for two hours at a time. Leave the bandage or compress intact. Simply keep the cloth cold. The first thing you will notice is an intensification of the itching, and/or pain. Continue treatment despite this. Beneficial reactions will soon begin to set in. Itching and pain will subside. Repeat twice daily for a week or as long as is necessary.

THE HOT WATER/SULFUR TECHNIQUE
FOR CHRONIC ECZEMA

STEPS TO TAKE:

1. HOT COMPRESS or HOT FOMENTS: treatment here is just the opposite of the treatment for the acute problem. Continue dousing the compress with hot water. Let it to remain on for 20 minutes. Follow removal of the hot pack with a cold water ablution. To do this pour cold water from a tea kettle or Scotch-douche it (spray).

2. DIETARY CONTROLS.
   A. Stick to a bland diet (cereals, vegetables, but NO MEAT!) If you like yoghurt or sour milk, add this to your diet.
   B. Plenty of liquids (fruit or vegetable juices).

3. OTHER CONTROLS.
   A. Get plenty of sleep.
   B. Cleanse the bowels with colonic irrigations (enema of warm water followed by cold water).

4. BRAN or SULFUR BATHS: (How to do them follows).

SULFUR EMOLLIENT BATH

To a tub filled two thirds with warm water, add five ounces of sulfurated lime or ten teaspoonsful of zinc sulfate crystals which you may pick up at the drug store. Make certain that all crystals are dissolved by swishing the water around and around. Keep the body-beautiful in the tub for only 20 minutes! Rise, pat dry, and permit a surface film of sulfur to remain. As a keratolytic and mild fungicide it will continue to do its job. This is an efficient method for many skin diseases as well as a procedure to stop chiggers. DO NOT use a follow-up shower! If you are allergic to sulfur DO NOT use this method.

BRAN EMOLLIENT BATH

Before bedtime here's the procedure: —Place two pounds of bran in a porous bag. Soak it in a pan of hot water for 20 minutes. By this time your full hot tub will be ready. Dump the pan of hot water and the bran bag right into the tub. Get in. Relax. After 15 minutes start massaging yourself all over with the bran bag. Keep mashing it against yourself. This leaves a sticky mess. Tub time is 20 minutes. Get out. *Pat*, don't rub, yourself dry. This will leave a sticky film all over you. With your bed previously prepared with plastic sheeting—above and beneath your body—go to bed and sleep. The next morning swish the bran film from your body. Note the gentle and fine texture of your skin after showering.

FEVERS . . . AND HOW
TO DOUSE THE FLAME

When fevers occur, the first thought usually is to lower it. This is not always the thing to do, however. There's a reason for fever. The heat of fever consumes bacterial invaders of the human body. Aspirin is usually administered and the discomfort of fever is admittedly alleviated. BUT, this does not get rid of the cause! To get rid of that cause by natural methods, water can be used to eliminate poisonous waste from the body and its parts. In all fever conditions, the reason for water therapy is to stimulate in some cases and sedate in other. In all cases, vital functions must be restored. The skin begins to do its own job and body temperature lowers. Blood vessels and nerves begin to function. Antibodies, antitoxins, phagocytes, etc. all go to work. They are all marshalled up by water therapy to do their job. With the body utilizing its own inborn natural processes, disease is countered.

How to Use Internal and
External Baths to
Conquer Fever

Despite the best of medical care, there are times when fevers continue no matter what the treatment administered. Where this problem exists water therapy—internally and externally—is the treatment of choice.

Quite often, just by cooling the abdomen, a fever will disappear. I have witnessed this happen time after time despite fevers of 103°-106°F. I remember one case of a youngster with a tense abdomen, sharp agonizing abdominal pain and all the earmarks of appendicitis.

The family doctor was on vacation. No one was covering for him. The family was desperate for help—any kind—even natural remedies, and they turned to me. The child was in agony. Fever—106°F and Dr. August Reingold's statement was still fresh in my mind—*"Cool the abdomen . . . conquer the fever!"*

Cold compresses were placed on the child's tummy after gentle manipulative pressures on the sore spots along the dorsal vertebrae. There were also zones of tenderness on his feet. Find these painful areas on your own feet and back. Apply pressure. You will jump and maybe yelp. Little Johnny K. did but I kept pressing anyhow. Slowly but surely he relaxed and went to sleep. I remained with the youngster through the night. When the fever went down, I put the family enema bag to work. After cleansing it with boiling water I filled it with cold water and added a tablespoonful of table salt. In cleansing the bowel with the solution I kept track of what was being voided. At first nothing appeared. Then a huge bolus—a big wad of waste—came out. I wondered how in the world he even managed to pass it. He yelled as it made its exit. He bled a little. But what was fantastic about it was that his bowels started to move. They moved and moved! His big hard belly went down. He didn't have appendicitis! What he'd had was a clogged colon and getting the cork out was all he needed.

STEPS TO TAKE:

1. COLD COMPRESSES on the abdomen as indicated above.

2. COLD INTESTINAL LAVAGE of enema (Review Figure 9).

3. NEPTUNE'S GIRDLE (Review Figure 32).

4. DRIPPING MANTLE may be used in place of "Neptune's Girdle." It is excellent for all illnesses with fever. It is especially good in child care for *scarlet fever, measles, chicken pox, mumps, diphtheria* and *influenza*.

Procedure:

Apply the "Dripping Mantle" in a warm room. To apply it,

wrap a sheet (soaked in cold water) around you. If you can't do it yourself, have a friend or relative apply it. Wrap fast. The sheet must make firm contact with the skin including the extremities. Stroke the cloth down tight to the skin. Just stand there in the bathtub. Keep the mantle on for three minutes. Remove and rub yourself glowingly dry and hop into a warm bed. This is not a pack. It is not a bath. It's a wet mantle and as such is one of the excellent water therapy procedures you can use in the home to cope with fever.

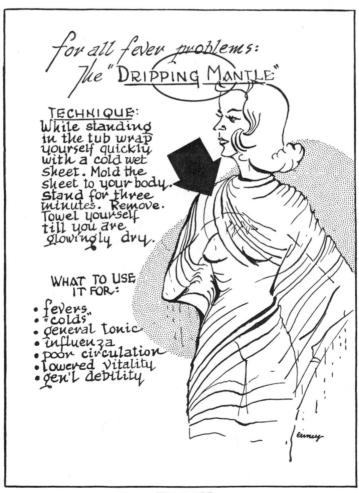

Figure 35

At-a-Glance
Information

Additional Illnesses That May
Be Treated with

THE DRIPPING MANTLE

Fevers (to decrease internal congestion)

Colds (to accentuate sweating and elimination
of toxic waste through the skin

General debility

Autointoxification (self-poisoning)

Lowered vitality

General tonic

Poor circulation

Influenza

ADDITIONAL HOME PROCEDURES
FOR TREATING FEVER
WITH WATER THERAPY

5. HOT PACKS may be given wet or dry. Their purpose is
to induce opening of the pores and induce sweating. It is easily
accomplished by wrapping the blanket around yourself or the
patient. The blanket is warmed—if to be applied dry—in an oven
or near a fireplace. If it is to be applied wet, it may be soaked in a
bathtub full of hot water. Over-wrap either the wet or dry blanket
with other dry blankets. Maintain the blanket wrap on an average
of a half hour while sitting in a comfortable chair. Administer
cool drinks. Keep an ice bag on your head. After the hot pack is
removed, rub the entire body and limbs with a coarse towel or
mitten. Go to bed. Sleep!

6. SECTIONAL ABLUTIONS may be given where the full bath is not possible in the treatment of fever. Sponge sections of the extremities and body one at a time with hot water. Follow immediately with cold sponging. Repeat four times daily. You will note that as the effect sets in you will have less and less desire to urinate because the skin is evacuating a large amount of watery waste. Keep the balance of the body covered as you expose each part for sponging. You may drink fruit juices during the process. To this excellent method, I suggest that hot and cold compresses be placed over the kidney areas. Alternate them. Follow with a hot water enema. This is one of the most effective methods I now for children's diseases such as scarlet fever, mumps, chicken pox, measles, etc.

7. COLD COMPRESSES for the throat may be used where complications—from some fever illness—have set in. Utilize a large turkish towel folded in fourths lengthwise. Soak in cold water. Wrap around the throat. Keep renewing the wrap as it warms. Repeat for 30 minutes. If you want to get a relaxing effect from it, alternate the compresses hot and cold. Time: Ten minutes hot. Five minutes cold. End with cold.

SPECIAL NOTE:

A. *Between baths of any kind, where there is fever, keep cold compresses over the area of the heart. Maintain this for 20 to 30 minutes.*

B. *Repeat all water therapies for one week AFTER RECOVERY! This builds resistance and copes with the after-effects. Bathe morning and afternoon and before bedtime.*

C. *AVOID CHILLING under all circumstances!*

A BETTER WAY TO BEAT
HEAT PROSTRATION

It was spring-workout time. Football, no less, and the heat was unbearable on the field. Although the players were not in full gear, the sun was taking its toll. Jimmy S. was the first to succumb. In laying him out in the shade, I found him breathing fast, his pulse faint. He was weak, dizzy, nauseated. His skin was pale and cool, but all such signs must not be interpreted as "sunstroke." Although the person having the problem should be placed in a cool shady place—as in sunstroke—the similarity stops there. For anyone knocked out by the heat—including athletes—the following procedure is great: —

STEPS TO TAKE:

1. REST IN A COOL SHADY PLACE.

2. HOT DRINKS immediately to stimulate the heart and activate the sweat glands.

3. FULL NEUTRAL BATH (90°-95°F) for 20 minutes with friction-rub. If a bathtub is not available, simply rub the skin with hot water. Rub, rub, rub. Massage for ten minutes. Follow the heat application with cold. Repeat both procedures daily for ten minutes until fully recovered.

4. NO FOOD!

5. CRACKED ICE and GINGER ALE may be taken orally ON THE SECOND DAY! No milk products! Thin soup (broth) and crackers are permitted.

SUNSTROKE
and Water Magic That Cures It

It is wise to know how to differentiate *sunstroke* from *heat prostration* because each has its own distinctive treatment. To simplify the matter for you, I am repeating the signs of heat prostration so that you may compare them with sunstroke. Remember in the knowing and in the understanding, comes success through water therapy. By using Nature's remedies you solve the problem that has ended in disaster for those who do not have this understanding or procedure.

SUNSTROKE:

Sunstroke comes on suddenly. The face gets flushed, hot, the pulse is fast and sometimes weak, breathing gets difficult and even noisy. Unconsciousness may result. Temperature may shoot up to 108°F. Remember that *sunstroke ALWAYS OCCURS IN THE SUN*! It does not occur in closed quarters!

HEAT PROSTRATION:

Heat prostration starts with a feeling of weakness or even unconsciousness. The face and skin are cool, pale, may show a cold sweat. Breathing is hastened. The pulse is stepped up. Body temperature goes *below* normal. This problem in most part is confined to hot quarters but may be due to the sun or on a muggy day. Study this differentiation closely. The life you save may be your own.

STEPS TO TAKE:

1. COLD ABLUTIONS may be applied—body part by body part with cold water friction or rubbing with ice. In either method the rubbing must continue for several hours or until such time as the temperature goes down and the signs and symptoms have disappeared.

2. COLD COMPRESS must be placed immediately over the heart and on the head. Replace the compress every five minutes or earlier if it is heating.

3. SCOTCH DOUCHE cold water spray (if bathtub or shower room is available). Continue showering until rectal temperature drops to 100°F. At this point, get into bed. Place cold compresses on the head, heart area and abdomen. Change these compresses every 30 minutes or less.

4. ENVIRONMENT should be a cool shady room with good ventilation.

SPECIAL NOTES:

1. Do NOT use an ice bath!

2. Baldheaded people should cover their heads when in the sun. Dr. Kley and I were fishing one summer in Pennsylvania. We were walking with waders downstream when he keeled over. I checked him out in the water. It was sunstroke. I left him lying there in the cold stream. His recovery was rapid.

water

treatment

for

MISCELLANEOUS

AILMENTS

---

chapter

10

Subjects covered:

Blood Pressure
Insomnia
Overweight (obesity)

HIGH BLOOD PRESSURE
And How to Handle It At Home

Tree Surgeon Finds Relief
From High Blood Pressure
Through Water Therapy

Ever had a feeling of tiredness, nervousness, dizziness, and inside your chest your heart was going bang, bang, bang? Ever had feelings of weakness, sleeplessness, and had all this accompanied by headaches? While all this was going on did you have the desire to vomit? Eyelids feel heavy? Did your usual nice personality change to not-so-nice? While this was going on did you get pains in your chest or have to get up from bed a dozen times each night to urinate? Did your nose bleed for reasons unknown?

Well if any of this has ever happened to you you'll know what tree surgeon George G. was going through when he presented himself in my office and reported exactly all this. Upon examination, I found that George was no world-beater. Obviously he was an average guy working for average wages. With what was happening to him it looked as though he wouldn't even be working for wages anymore unless his problem was corrected. He told me how doctors had him on drugs and that he was walking around like a zombie under tranquilizers. He said he had learned his blood pressure was 220 over 140 and getting progressively worse. He admitted that he was scared. That was his word for it—"scared." I could see that what George needed most—before any kind of treatment began—was reassurance. He had to be helped. Today, George looks, feels and acts like a new man. Even his blood pressure is under control.

In presenting the program necessary for his recovery I laid out the following—

STEPS TO TAKE:

1. PROLONGED NEUTRAL BATH, daily, one to three hours at 90°-95°F. Keep a cold compress on your head during the entire bath.

2. HOT FOOT and LEG BATH may be accomplished with a bucket or while sitting on the edge of the bathtub spraying your extremities. A more highly effective procedure is to stand in a bathtub full of hot water while spraying up and down the spine with cold water. Treatment time is ten minutes.

3. HOT COMPRESSES over the heart should be re-applied as they cool down. Rub the skin with olive oil before applying the hot pack. Overlay the pack with a plastic bib to maintain the heat. Lie there and rest. One, or all, of these methods may be used per day. For immediate effectiveness I recommend Step Two followed by the *"Million-Dollar Carotid Sinus Technique."*

Here, Now, Is that "Million-Dollar Carotid Sinus Technique" for Blood Pressure

CAROTID SINUS . . . MILLION-DOLLAR CONTROL TOWER

First, go back and review Figure 24. What is the *carotid sinus*? The carotid sinus is a ductless gland (no outlets). One is located on each side of the neck as part of the carotid artery and is easily accessible. You have only to reach up and there it is.

Exactly where? As a reminder, here's how to find it and what to do to help yourself if you have high blood pressure and need to use that million-dollar control tower right now.

Step One:

Locate the top of your Adam's apple. Slide your fingers backward on each side of your throat till you come to a pulse. That's it! Here lies the million-dollar carotid sinus and you're in the driver's seat for controlling it. Remember that this very important gland on each side of your neck regulates blood pressure up and down. It is connected with special nerve-end organs that cause high blood pressure to happen. And because of its direct connection with a magic part of the brain called the *medulla oblongata*, it can increase and decrease the heart rate on demand. Press this amazing control button semi-hard. Just once! ONE time per day ONLY! Then go on to the next step. (REMEMBER: press the "button" ONLY ONCE!)

Step Two:

Along with the carotid sinus, there are two more important points to be contacted with your finger tips. One is on the top of the head. It's dead center on the crown. Locate it right now. Here you will find an area of exquisite tenderness in the scalp—at its midline—if you are having a true blood pressure problem. (*Note:* this same point will be extremely tender if you have hemorrhoids which often accompany changes in blood pressure.) Sometimes this scalp area is so tender you can't run a comb through your hair.

Now take the finger tips of both hands and place them in this area. Place your thumbs on the bony bump (mastoid process) behind each ear. Take a firm grip and maintain the grasp as you move the scalp forward and back on your skull. Note also how tender this area behind the mastoid process is. All of these are extremely important nerve centers that no knowledgeable person will pooh-pooh aside. They are "buttons" in your control tower! Use them effectively!

Step Three:

Locate the bony ridge at the base and back of your skull. Note the many small areas of distress as your fingertips probe along this ridge. Apply pressure on each. Make tiny rotary motions on each for a slow ten count. Repeat the procedure at least three times and at no time be rough in your treatment.

Step Four:

Now get the tips of the third finger on each hand into the hollow at the base of the skull. Compress. Make tiny rotary motions with your fingertips until the pain is gone. The very fact that the tenderness is leaving will attest to the fact that your treatment is actively at work inside.

Step Five:

Place the fingertips of both hands into the area just below the tip of the breastbone. Expel all air from your lungs. Apply pressure with your fingers on this area. Hold for a slow five count and release. Breathe. Repeat three times.

Step Six:

In this final step, wrap your throat with a cold wet towel. (The towel should be folded lengthwise in fourths.) Saturate with cold water. Squeeze out the excess water. Repeat the process as the wrap warms. Now place an ice bag on your solar plexus area, lie back and relax. In just moments you will begin to experience a pleasurably relaxed warm feeling. Let go! Relax! Twenty minutes of this and you'll be ready to go once more. I know! When everything else failed that's what I applied on myself for high blood pressure and found relief.

LOW BLOOD PRESSURE PROBLEMS
And What You Can Do About Them

Al K. had *low blood pressure*. He complained that he was always feeling tired, that he was wornout and couldn't concentrate on his job. What he had wasn't much of a job but it was all that Al could hold down under the circumstance. He came back from the Vietnam war feeling mighty low. No wounds, no bad habits or disease picked up over there. It was just that "zipped out" feeling. After he got nowhere at the military hospitals, he started making the rounds of local physicians. Everyone of his doctors spotted the low blood pressure problem immediately. He told them about his headaches and about the tight feeling in his chest. He told them about how his heart fluttered and that he simply pooped out no matter what he did. He was put on medications and told to rest. But how could he rest? He had a job to hold down. He had to take care of his Mom and Dad. Both were sick and couldn't get around much anymore. It was a problem and the complications aggravated his low blood pressure.

I couldn't find anything wrong with what these excellent physicians were doing for Al. In fact, I concurred with their treatment and diagnosis. He had low blood pressure all right but as far as I was concerned these symptoms were merely warning signals. I believed Al to be in relatively good shape except for lazy heart muscles that needed to be stepped up in their duties. I felt that when the blood started circulating the dizziness would go away. His mind would become clear. He would be alert once more and this is exactly what happened!

If you have ever had low blood pressure from any cause you will want to use my method of stimulating the "Million-Dollar Carotid Sinus Technique," and when you use it—if you truly have low blood pressure resulting from an inactive heart—you will find the treatment truly worth a million dollars to you.

What to Do About Low Blood Pressure

STEPS TO TAKE:

1. COLD SHOWER BATHS of short duration are used to stimulate the peripheral circulation (blood vessels under the skin) and act reflexly on all organs of the abdomen and chest. Because of this stimulation, metabolism (body function) is stepped up and blood pressure *increases*. This means keeping one thought in mind—*"Use the cold shower for raising your blood pressure BUT ONLY FOR A FEW SECONDS!"* Remember, short cold treatments stimulate. Prolonged cold therapy sedates. Nature will take over and do the job that has to be done!

2. ICE BAGS over the heart for 15 to 30 minutes not only slow the pulse, but raise the blood pressure. Place a damp face cloth down before placing the ice bag. Now and again lift the ice bag. Rub the skin with tepid water. In this case, prolonged ice application over this area produces wonderful reflex actions of Nature in distant parts of the body. Circulating blood is cooled. (*Note:* Do not permit the skin to become blanched (pale or white). Another version of the ice procedure I have used is called the "Heart Coil." If you are sufficiently mechanical minded, you can accomplish it with nothing more than the rubber hose from your enema bag coiled over the heart area. With the outlet tube running into a bucket beside the bed turn on the cut-off valve to permit ice water to flow through *slowly*. I advocate this coil technique because it improves the nutrition to the heart wall by way of stimulating the coronary arteries. Contractions slow down in the heart muscle. Because of this I find this treatment also of value for pneumonia, diphtheria and severe fevers.

3. WATER DRINKING (hot or cold) increases blood pressure and reflexly controls contractions of the cardiac muscle.

FOR WOMEN ONLY

4. HOT VAGINAL DOUCHE (very hot) may be *used in an emergency where the blood pressure drops suddenly*. The hot douche is at first an excitant. Later, it becomes very relaxing and acts as a sedative. The effects derived are brief but vital in an emergency. Water temperature may be 110°-112°F. Raise the enema bag high so that the flow of water is fast and strong. Keep the nozzle in constant motion so that there is no concentrated collection of heat in one place.

5. Cerney's MILLION-DOLLAR CAROTID SINUS TECHNIQUE (Review Figure 24).

HOW TO CONQUER INSOMNIA
WITH WATER THERAPY

Insomnia in itself is not a disease. It is a symptom, however, of something wrong in the systems of the body as well as mind. It may be due to auto-intoxication (self-created poisoning), infections, constitutional diseases, overwork, sexual excitement, bedtime eating, consumption of alcohol, mental excitement, poor ventilation in the sleeping room or being just plain cold. To solve the problem, here is a method for releasing cerebral congestion that makes sleep impossible:—

STEPS TO TAKE:

1. WARM FULL BATH (90°-95°F) for 20 minutes. Lie in the tub submerged to the chin before bedtime. *DO NOT FOLLOW WITH A COLD SHOWER* or other cold applications.

2. COLD FOOT BATH or WATER TREADING may be achieved in the bathtub. Two other methods to accomplish the same effect are that of—(a) *cold compresses* with wet toweling

wrapped around the feet and legs, or (b) *Heavy sweat socks* dunked into and withdrawn from a bucket of cold water. In all these four methods, overwrap the foot and its dressing with a plastic sheet and remain in bed covered warmly.

3. COLD COMPRESSES on the abdomen should be changed as they warm. Repeat the process three times and go to sleep.

4. HOT LIQUIDS BY MOUTH before retiring may be milk, brandy, lemonade.

5. WELL-VENTILATED BEDROOM (cool air) with warm bed-clothing.

6. AUTO-SUGGESTION—tell yourself to relax as part of your self disciplining. Begin at the bottom and anatomically move up. Say each body part by name—"Feet, relax, let go. Legs, relax . . . let go," etc. to the top of the head. Keep repeating the process until you are well indoctrinated in self-command.

CAN OVERWEIGHT BE CORRECTED WITH THE MAGIC OF WATER THERAPY?

In a nation highly beauty-conscious such as the U.S.A., everyone thinks about "looking nice." As a result, losing weight to conform to the ideals of a "beautiful figure," has become a necessity. Under controlled circumstances, weight should, and can, be lost for health reasons as well as for beauty. In obesity there are a number of complicating factors of which to be aware.

Obesity occurs more often in women than in men and usually starts in the middle years of life. Although heredity is a possible cause, it is a rare one. The most common offender lies in habits and eating. Eating too much and moving around too little fails to consume the caloric intake. This lays up as fat, and fat, according to the physiologists and nutritionists, should be "burned in the fire of carbohydrates."

Since it is difficult for people to control their diet they have recourse to other measures. Therapy with cold water is such a measure, bringing about a warming reaction that helps in controlled-weight-loss. Why cold water for obesity? Cold water steps up metabolism! It re-energizes body processes leading back to health! As the body's energy centers begin to function, the fat is consumed. Digestion and absorption are improved. Glands (such as the thyroid) are stimulated. Glands, other than the thyroid (hypothalamus, ovaries, testes, pituitary) burn up fat.

There may be psychological reasons for obesity. Frustration, unhappiness, nervous tension may lead to the piling up of fat. For some folks becoming fat creates a weapon to fight others by demanding special attention and sympathy. Katherine S. was a good example of this. She was so much overweight she looked almost as wide as she was high.

As Katherine's weight grew so did the pain in her feet and knees. Her thighs and low back ached. In every crease her skin was macerated and odorous. She developed diabetes. Her blood pressure went up. She hated the world because she was no longer "pretty" and she couldn't be blamed for that. After a complete examination to rule out possible complications, I found Katherine's biggest problem to be psychological. Because she was afraid her husband didn't want her anymore she was eating her way into oblivion. She was simply "digging her own grave with her teeth."

In most part obesity is an acquired characteristic. Seldom inherited. Since it is acquired, the process can also be reversed. Before using any measure for "getting rid of weight" see your doctor. If he says you are physically fit, then you can use a procedure such as follows:—

STEPS TO TAKE:

1. BLANKET or TENT SITZ BATH is almost unknown in the U.S.A. and yet it is so simple to set up and use. (See Figure 36.) Its purpose is to promote sweating even as it decongests and stimulates all the digestive and pelvic organs. (It is excellent as a

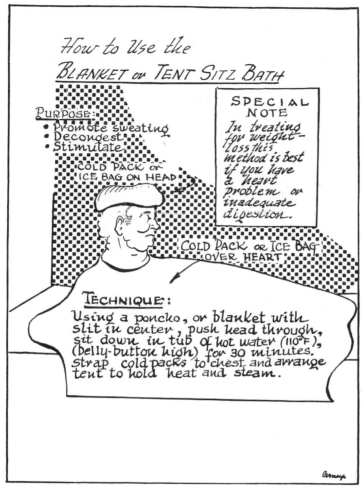

Figure 36

therapy for abdominal problems when one is not concerned about obesity.) The *tent sitz* is of especial value in weight reduction where the overweight is complicated by heart and digestive conditions that need attention. Because it is effective and gentle in inducing sweat, it is ideal for folks with these problems. How do you accomplish it? Lay four boards across the tub to keep the blanket from falling in. The blanket may be an old one with a hole to stick your head through in the center. It may be a Mexican poncho. With the water temperature at 105°-110°F, sit in water belly-button high for 15 to 30 minutes. End with a quick cold shower.

Maintain a cold pack on your head. Place another cold pack over your heart area. If you are a woman, stuff the cold pack under your brassiere to hold it in position. A man may utilize a pants belt. The method is safe and simple. After a brisk rub-down go to bed immediately. Sleep thee in peace.

2. COLD FULL or HALF BATH (70°-75°F) should be taken every other day for ten minutes at a time. Massage the entire body following this bath. Use active friction (see "Friction Rub") to step up skin activity and internal oxidation.

3. SPRAY TECHNIQUE or SCOTCH DOUCHE may be used with cold water applied *only* to the *lower half* of the body *each morning*. Spray cold water on the *upper half before bedtime each night*. As the spray hits, rub yourself briskly. Do this until warmth is obviously flowing in. Then proceed to the next area. *Note:* Two factors of importance—(a) if you have varicose veins on your legs and thighs DO NOT use the spray. DO NOT apply massage or rubbing! (b) If you have a cardiac (heart) problem DO NOT use this therapy.

4. FULL RELAXING BATH (Review Figure 16) is also highly efficient in the weight-loss routine. For persons like Katherine S., whose obesity began with mental turmoil and tensions, the relaxing bath works magic. Her general attitude changed about everything! Morale improved. Katherine got a whole new lease on life. Not only that! She went from 240 pounds down to 152 and it was the happiest day of her life to see what the scales registered. It was magic! Inside that butter ball was a lovely woman. After her skin contracted and the sags retreated, she started taking dancing lessons at Arthur Murray's. Her husband fell in love with her all over again and they lived happily every after.

5. REGULAR CONTROLLED EXERCISE PROGRAM should be worked out on a daily basis. This should include (in

season) swimming, golfing, bike riding, "health club activity", dancing, walking, etc. anything and everything to improve muscle tone, burn calories and build resistance as well as develop general good health.

6. DIETARY CONTROLS Check your family doctor first and have a complete physical examination. DO NOT go into a crash program! All of them end in some form of disaster. Stick to your doctor's suggested food control program. Remember, you are fat only in direct proportion to the food you consume. Your doctor, if he's on his toes, will recommend a diet high in proteins and low in fats. He will probably suggest low carbohydrates, bulky fruits and vegetables, and supplementary vitamins and minerals to make up for the insipid burned out foods we eat today.

In getting rid of obesity or overweight, you need more than a desire. You need to follow the rules of weight reduction. Stick to your doctor's rules. Stick to the hydrotherapy procedures so vital to weight loss and step by step—just as did Katherine S.—you will achieve the shapeliness you desire. It's within your power to do so. All you have to do is DO IT!

INDEX